Chronic Kidney Disease
A practical guide to
understanding and management

Chronic Kidney Disease
A practical guide to understanding and management

Edited by

Meguid El Nahas
Professor of Nephrology
Sheffield Kidney Institute
Sheffield, UK

and

Adeera Levin
Professor of Medicine
University of British Columbia
Consultant Nephrologist
Providence Health Care/St Paul's Hospital
Canada

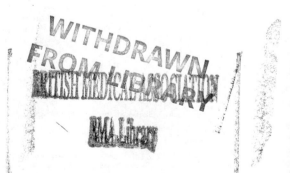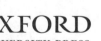
OXFORD
UNIVERSITY PRESS

OXFORD

UNIVERSITY PRESS

Great Clarendon Street, Oxford ox2 6dp

Oxford University Press is a department of the University of Oxford.
It furthers the University's objective of excellence in research, scholarship,
and education by publishing worldwide in

Oxford   New York

Auckland   Cape Town   Dar es Salaam   Hong Kong   Karachi
Kuala Lumpur   Madrid   Melbourne   Mexico City   Nairobi
New Delhi   Shanghai   Taipei   Toronto

With offices in

Argentina   Austria   Brazil   Chile   Czech Republic   France   Greece
Guatemala   Hungary   Italy   Japan   Poland   Portugal   Singapore
South Korea   Switzerland   Thailand   Turkey   Ukraine   Vietnam

Oxford is a registered trade mark of Oxford University Press
in the UK and in certain other countries

Published in the United States
by Oxford University Press Inc., New York

© Oxford University Press, 2009

British Library Cataloguing in Publication Data

Data available

Library of Congress Cataloging in Publication Data

Chronic kidney disease : a practical guide to understanding and management /
[edited by] A. Meguid El Nahas & Adeera Levin.
    p. ; cm.
  Includes index.
  ISBN 978-0-19-954931-3 (alk. paper)
  1. Chronic renal failure. 2. Chronic renal failure—Treatment.
  I. El Nahas, A. Meguid. II. Levin, A. (Adeera)
  [DNLM: 1. Renal Insufficiency, Chronic—therapy. WJ 342 C5563 2010]
  RC918.R4C576 2010
  616.6'14—dc22

                                                              2009037723

Typeset in Minion by Glyph International, Bangalore, India
Printed in Great Britain
on acid-free paper by
MPG Books Group, Bodmin and King's Lynn

ISBN 978-0-19-954931-3

10 9 8 7 6 5 4 3 2 1

Preface

Chronic kidney disease (CKD) has recently been established as an important condition affecting a significant percentage of the population. It usually affects those with cardiovascular disease (CVD), diabetes, and specific ethnic groups. It is also associated with the aging process in conjunction with accumulated comorbidities. The increasing awareness of the condition, ease of diagnosis with various laboratory initiative reporting estimated glomerular filtration rate (eGFR), and the rising prevalence and incidence of CVD and diabetes in the general population has made the understanding and treatment of kidney disease all the more important in this millennium. We have learned much about factors important in CKD susceptibility and progression as well as treatment options. There continues to be much more to learn. Nonetheless, early identification and treatment of common conditions such as hypertension, diabetes, and CVD risk reduction remain the cornerstone of therapy.

Chronic kidney disease: a practical guide to understanding and management is intended for the practising clinician, general, and nephrology house staff. The contributions from an international panel of experts in the field of CKD will help the clinician to gain a broad understanding of kidney disease, its treatments, and its attendant comorbidities. The global perspective portrayed in this book ensures its applicability across multiple jurisdictions, which we trust the readers will find useful.

We are indebted to all the authors for their valuable contributions to the book and for ensuring that the information is current and practical.

Overall, given the increasing identification of patients with kidney disease and our understanding of the importance of kidney function in the maintenance of health, this handbook provides valuable insights for the care of patients.

We hope that the readers will find the information provided herein helpful in the care of patients with CKD.

M El Nahas
A Levin

To all those who are affected, personally, socially
or professionally by chronic kidney disease

Contents

List of Contributors

Aimun Ahmed
Consultant
Nephrologist
Preston Renal Unit
Preston, UK

Marcellus Assiago
Staff Nephrologist
Iron Mission Dialysis Unit
Division of Nephrology
University of Utah
Salt Lake City, Utah

Robert C. Atkins
Head of Kidney Disease
Prevention, Department of
Epidemiology and Preventive
Medicine, Monash University
Victoria, Australia

Rashad Barsoum
Emeritus Professor of Medicine
Kasr-El-Aini Medical School
Cairo University
Egypt

Monica Beaulieu
Clinical Assistant Professor
St. Paul's Hospital
University of British Columbia
Canada

Neil Boudville
Senior Lecturer in Renal
Medicine

University of Western Australia
Consultant Nephrologist
Sir Charles Gairdner Hospital
Australia

Mohsen El Kossi
Consultant Nephrologist
Doncaster Renal Unit
Doncaster, UK

Meguid El Nahas
Professor of Nephrology
Sheffield Kidney Institute
Sheffield, UK

Jagbir Gill
Assistant Professor
St. Paul's Hospital
University of British Columbia
Canada

Kevin Harris
Consultant Nephrologist
John Walls Renal Unit
Leicester General Hospital
Leicester, UK

Fairol H. Ibrahim
Specialist Registrar in Nephrology
Sheffield Kidney Institute
Sheffield, UK

Bisher Kawar
Specialist Registrar in Nephrology
Sheffield Kidney Institute
Sheffield, UK

Andrew S.H. Lai
Resident Medical Officer
Department of Medicine
Queen Mary Hospital
The University of Hong Kong
Hong Kong

Kar Neng Lai
Yu Chiu Kwong Chair
of Internal Medicine, Chief of
Medicine
Department of Medicine
Queen Mary Hospital
The University of Hong Kong
Hong Kong

Andrew S. Levey
Chief, Divison of Nephrology
and Professor of Medicine
Tufts Medical Center
Boston, US

Adeera Levin
Professor of Medicine
University of British Columbia
Consultant Nephrologist
Providence Health Care/
St Paul's Hospital
Canada

Rakesh Patel
Specialist Registrar in Nephrology
John Walls Renal Unit
Leicester General Hospital
Leicester, UK

Anne T. Reutens
Consultant Endocrinologist/
Research Fellow
Baker IDI Heart and Diabetes
Institute, Department of
Epidemiology and Preventive
Medicine, Monash University
Victoria, Australia

Mark J. Sarnak
Associate Professor of Medicine
Tufts University School of
Medicine, Nephrologist
Tufts Medical Center
Boston, US

Lesley A. Stevens
Assistant Professor of Medicine
Tufts Medical Center
Boston, US

Sydney C.W. Tang
Associate Professor
Department of Medicine
Queen Mary Hospital
The University of Hong Kong
Hong Kong

Daniel E. Weiner
Associate Professor of Medicine
Tufts University School of
Medicine, Nephrologist
Tufts Medical Center
Boston, US

Abbreviations

>	greater than
<	less than
≥	equal to and greater than
~	approximately
α	alpha
β	beta
γ	gamma
κ	kappa
°C	degree Celsius
AASK	African American Study of Kidney disease and hypertension
AASV	ANCA-associated systemic vasculitis
ABCD	Appropriate Blood Pressure Control in Diabetes trial
ACCORD	Action to Control CardiOvascular Risk in Diabetes trial
ACEi	angiotensin-converting enzyme inhibitor
ACR	albumin-to-creatinine ratio
ADA	American Diabetes Association
ADPKD	autosomal dominant polycystic kidney disease
AI	augmentation index
AN	associated nephropathy
ANCA	anti-neutrophil cytoplasmic antibody
ANZDATA	Australia and New Zealand Dialysis and Transplant Registry
APD	automated peritoneal dialysis
APOE	apolipoprotein E
ARB	angiotensin II receptor blocker
ARIC	Atherosclerosis Risk In Communities
ARVD	atherosclerotic renal vascular disease
ATN	acute tubular necrosis
AV	arteriovenous
BCGPAC	British Columbia Guidelines and Protocols Advisory Committee
BHS	British Hypertension Society
BKV	Polyoma virus BK
BMI	body mass index
BNF	British National Formulary
BP	blood pressure
CAPD	chronic ambulatory peritoneal dialysis
CARI	Caring for Australians with Renal Impairment
CCB	calcium channel blockers
CCPD	continuous cycler-assisted peritoneal dialysis
cfu	colony-forming unit
CG	Cockroft–Gault
CHD	coronary heart disease
CHS	Cardiovascular Health Study
CI	confidence interval
CIC	circulating immune complexes
CK	creatine kinase
CKD	chronic kidney disease
CKD-MBD	chronic kidney disease-mineral and bone disorder
CK-MB	creatine kinase-MB
cm	centimetre
CMV	cytomegalovirus

CNI	calcineurin inhibitor	FSGS	focal segmental glomerulosclerosis
COX	cyclooxygenase	g	gram
CPG	clinical practice guideline	GBM	glomerular basement membrane
CSN	Canadian Society of Nephrology	GDP	gross domestic product per capita
CT	computed tomography	GFR	glomerular filtration rate
CVD	cardiovascular disease	GN	glomerulonephritis
DASH	Dietary Approaches to Stop Hypertension	GP	general practitioner
DCCT	Diabetes Control and Complications Trial	h	hour
DBP	diastolic blood pressure	Hb	haemoglobin
DEXA	dual-energy X-ray absorptiometry	HBeAg	hepatitis B e antigen
		HBsAg	hepatitis B surface antigen
DKD	diabetic kidney disease	HBV	hepatitis B virus
dL	decilitre	HCV	hepatitis C virus
DM	diabetes mellitus	HD	haemodialysis
DN	diabetic nephropathy	HDL	high density lipoprotein
DNA	deoxyribonucleic acid	HHV	human herpesvirus
DOPPS	Dialysis Outcomes and Practice Patterns study	HIV	human immunodeficiency virus
DRC	Democratic Republic of Congo	HIV-AN	HIV-associated nephropathy
DRVD	Diabetic renal vascular disease	HOT	Hypertension Optimal Treatment
EBPG	European Best Practice Guidelines for the management of hypertension	HPV	human papillomavirus
		HR	hazard ratio
		HSP	Henoch–Schönlein purpura
ECG	electrocardiography	HUS/TTP	haemolytic-uraemic syndrome/thrombotic thrombocytopaenic purpura
ED	emergency department		
e.g.	*exempli gratia*; for example		
eGFR	estimated glomerular filtration rate	IC	immune complexes
		ICD	implantable cardioverter defibrillator
ERA-EDTA	European Renal Association–European Dialysis and Transplant Association	IDNT	Irbesartan in Diabetic Nephropathy Trial
		i.e.	*id est*; that is
ESA	erythropoietin-stimulating agent	Ig	immunoglobulin
		IgAN	IgA nephropathy
ESRD	end-stage renal disease	ISN	International Society of Nephrology
ESRF	end-stage renal failure		
FGF	fibroblast growth factor	IU	international units

IV	intravenous	NICE	National Institute for Health and Clinical Excellence
IVU	intravenous urogram		
KDIGO	Kidney Disease: Improving Global Outcomes	NIDDM	non-insular dependent diabetes mellitus
KDOQI	Kidney Disease Outcomes Quality Initiative	NKF	National Kidney Foundation
KEEP	Kidney Early Evaluation program	NSAID	non-steroidal anti-inflammatory drug
kg	kilogram	NT-proBNP	N-terminal pro-B-type natriuretic peptide
km	kilometre	ONTARGET	ONgoing Telmisartan Alone and in combination with Ramipril Global Endpoint Trial
L	litre		
lb	pound		
LDL	low density lipoprotein		
LV	left ventricle	OR	odds ratio
LVH	left ventricular hypertrophy	p	probability
		PCP	primary care physician; *Pneumocystis carinii* pneumonia
m	metre		
MA	microalbuminuria		
MAP	mean arterial pressure	PCR	protein-to-creatinine ratio
MCD	minimal change disease	PD	peritoneal dialysis
MCGN	mesangiocapillary glomerulonephritis	PHS	Physicians' Health Study
		PICC	peripherally inserted central catheter
MDC	multidisciplinary clinic		
MDRD	Modification of Diet in Renal Disease study	pmp	per million population
		PP	pulse pressure
mg	milligram	PREVEND	Prevention of Renal and Vascular End-stage Disease
μg	microgram		
min	minute		
mL	millilitre	PSGN	post-streptococcal glomerulonephritis
MMF	mycophenolate mofetil	PTH	parathyroid hormone
mmHg	millimetre mercury	PV	parvovirus
mmol	millimole	PWV	pulse wave velocity
MN	membranous nephropathy	QALY	quality-adjusted life year
MPGN	mesangioproliferative glomerulonephritis	RAAS	renin-angiotensin-aldosterone system
MR	magnetic resonance	RCT	randomized controlled trial
MRFIT	Multiple Risk Factor Intervention Trial		
mRNA	messenger ribonucleic acid	REIN	Ramipril Efficacy in Nephropathy
NHANES	National Health and Nutrition Examination Surveys	REGARDS	Reasons for Geographic and Racial Differences in Stroke) Cohort Study

RENAAL	Reduction of Endpoints in NIDDM with the Angiotensin II Antagonist Losartan
RF	rheumatoid factors
RR	relative risk
RRT	renal replacement therapy
SARS	severe acute respiratory syndrome
SBP	systolic blood pressure
SCUF	slow continuous ultrafiltration
SEM	standard error of the mean
SGA	subjective global assessment
SNS	sympathetic nervous system
SLE	systemic lupus erythematosus
TIBC	total iron binding capacity
TNF	tumour necrosis factor
UAE	urine albumin excretion
UK	United Kingdom
UKPDS	United Kingdom Prospective Diabetes Study
US	United States
USRDS	US Renal Data System
USS	ultrasound scanning
UTI	urinary tract infection
vs	versus
y	year

Chapter 1

Practical approaches to the diagnosis and management of common nephrological problems

Bisher Kawar, Mohsen El Kossi, Rakesh Patel, Kevin Harris, and Meguid El Nahas

This introductory chapter outlines practical diagnostic and management approaches to common nephrological problems frequently encountered in primary care. These include proteinuria, haematuria, hypertension and urinary tract infections. Also included in this chapter is a brief description of the nephrologist's approach to glomerulonephritis and diabetic nephropathy, two of the most common causes of chronic kidney disease (CKD). This is aimed at informing primary care physicians and non-nephrologists of diagnostic and prognostic approaches to these conditions and also highlighting different aspects of their management. The chapter also includes guidance to the use of drugs/medication in patients with CKD. It is hoped that this introductory chapter will assist those dealing with a range of common nephrological presentations in primary care. Subsequent chapters in the handbook address in more details specific topics related to CKD.

Practical approach to proteinuria

Introduction

Proteinuria is one of the main manifestations of kidney disease. In this context, it mainly refers to albuminuria. Non-albumin proteinuria, which is not detectable by conventional 'dipstick' analysis such as

Table 1.1 Terminology and definitions of albuminuria and proteinuria

Proteinuria	Generic term used to describe the presence of protein in urine. Usually refers to 'dipstick'-detectable proteinuria which is likely to be albumin at a concentration of >300mg/L.
Albuminuria	A term specific to the presence of albumin in the urine and should only be used when confirmed by a laboratory immunoassay.
Microalbuminuria	Urine albumin excretion rate of 30–300mg/24h.
Macroalbuminuria	Urine albumin excretion rate of >300mg/24h.
Nephrotic range proteinuria	Proteinuria >3.5g/24h.
Nephrotic syndrome	Nephrotic range proteinuria with a syndrome of oedema, serum hypoalbuminaemia, hyperlipidaemia, and thrombophilia.

$\beta2$ microglobulin and immunoglobulins, is beyond the scope of this chapter. The definition of CKD stages 1 and 2 most often refers to individuals with proteinuria and a glomerular filtration rate >60mL/min/ 1.73m^2. Therefore, it is important to be familiar with proteinuria, its terminology, detection methods as well as clinical implications and management.

Proteinuria is often asymptomatic below at least 3g/24h when it could present as frothy urine or oedema. Different terms are used when describing proteinuria. Those are summarized in Table 1.1.

Detection and measurement of proteinuria

Conventional reagent strip or 'dipstick' analysis is based on a colorimetric indicator (bromocresol green) which changes colour in the presence of protein. It can detect an albumin concentration of around 300mg/L. An arbitrary scale of +1 to +4 based on the intensity of the colour change gives an indication of the concentration of protein which roughly corresponds to <0.5g for +1 and >1g for +3/+4, though this is far from accurate. Therefore, in clinical practice, this should be confirmed by laboratory quantification. Causes of false positive and false negative results are summarized in Table 1.2.

Table 1.2 Causes of false positive and false negative reagent strip test for proteinuria

Causes of false positive	Causes of false negative
Heavily alkaline urine (pH >8)	Positively charged proteins, e.g. tubular proteins, Bence–Jones protein.
Dehydration causing increased concentration	Excessive hydration causing dilution and low concentration.
Transient increase in urinary protein excretion: exercise, infection	
Haematuria	
Drugs, e.g. penicillin, cephalosporins, miconazole	
Contrast medium	

Rationale for laboratory quantification

Quantifying proteinuria is essential in clinical practice for the following reasons:

- To determine the diagnostic nature of CKD: it gives an indication of the nature of kidney disease. Diseases of glomerular origin tend to be associated with higher levels of proteinuria than tubulointerstitial or vascular diseases. Within the glomerular disease, certain conditions are more likely to present with nephrotic range proteinuria such as minimal change disease, focal and segmental glomerulosclerosis, and membranous nephropathy; whilst others such as mesangioproliferative conditions are likely to present with subnephrotic range proteinuria (see 'Practical approach to glomerulonephritis').

- To determine the prognosis of kidney disease: the degree of proteinuria is one of the major determinants of the progression of CKD.

- Proteinuria is also associated with poor cardiovascular disease outcomes (CVD).

- To monitor progression/regression of CKD and response to treatment: regression of proteinuria can be the first sign of response to treatment. This may be partial or complete. Similarly, increase or reappearance of proteinuria can be the first sign of a relapse.

Tests to quantify proteinuria

Tests to qualify proteinuria are summarized in Table 1.3.

There is evidence that measurements of urine protein-to-creatinine ratio (PCR) or albumin-to-creatinine ratio (ACR) in a first morning void gives the best estimate for 24h excretion and is superior to random/spot urine sampling.

Protein vs albumin

Urinary protein refers to total protein which includes albumin and the so-called tubular proteins. Therefore, it is invariably higher than urinary albumin. However, for the majority of kidney diseases, especially those of glomerular origin, most of the urine protein is albumin (~60%)

Table 1.3 Proteinuria testing

Test	Rationale	Advantages	Disadvantages
24h urine collection	A direct measurement of protein or albumin excretion rate.	A true measurement of protein excretion in 24h rather than an estimation and therefore, considered the gold standard.	Inconvenient to patients. Inaccurate collections.
Protein or albumin concentration	An indication of protein excretion from a spot urine sample.	More convenient than 24h collection. Gives a reasonable indication of degree of proteinuria.	Concentration depends on urine volume and hydration status. Protein excretion is not constant during the day.
Protein- or albumin-to-creatinine ratio (PCR or ACR)	Correcting albumin concentration for creatinine eliminates the volume effect as creatinine excretion is assumed to be constant.	Convenient to patients. Can be used to estimate 24h excretion, e.g. by multiplying by 10 if expressed in mg/mmol	Is only an estimate of 24h excretion. The multiplication factor, e.g. 10, assumes a creatinine excretion rate of 10mmol/24h. This is only true for an average build. Cannot be used in a situation where creatinine excretion is rapidly changing, e.g. acute kidney injury, catabolic state.

and either measurement could be used. Depending on the place of practice, measurement of total protein is usually cheaper than measuring albumin and tends to be the main reason for using it in preference to albumin. In any case, when monitoring disease activity or progression, it is best to use the same measurement. Recently, in the UK, new National Institute for Health and Clinical Excellence (NICE) CKD guidelines have recommended measurement of urine ACR in preference to PCR due to its higher specificity. The conversion suggested for switching between measurements is 70mg/mmol protein equivalent to 50mg/mmol albumin.

Clinical significance of proteinuria

In the general population, a number of risk factors have been associated in cohort studies with the development of proteinuria. These include age, obesity, smoking as well as dyslipidaemia. A large body of literature attributes to proteinuria/albuminuria significant prognostic values in the general population and patients with CKD. In the former, this is primarily related to poor CVD outcomes whilst in CKD patients, proteinuria is a reliable marker of CKD progression (see Chapter 3). The level of proteinuria also guides the management of hypertensive patients with CKD; patients with high levels of proteinuria (>1g/24h) are preferentially treated with inhibitors of the renin-angiotensin-aldosterone system (RAAS).

Microalbuminuria

Over the last 25 years, microalbuminuria has been considered the forerunner of overt proteinuria in patients with diabetic nephropathy. However, a considerable percentage of diabetic people with low level microalbuminuria 30–150mg/24h do not progress to overt proteinuria and even reverse back to normoalbuminuria upon control of risk factors such as hyperglycaemia, hypertension, and dyslipidaemia.

In the general population, microalbuminuria has been considered a parameter to diagnose CKD (stages 1 and 2). A number of population-based studies have revealed a prevalence of microalbuminuria of around 6–7% (see Chapter 4). However, it is important to appreciate that microalbuminuria is not specific to kidney disease as it is elevated in a

Table 1.4 Factors influencing microalbuminuria

Physiological	Exercise
	High protein diet
Glomerular pathology	Early glomerulonephritis
	Early diabetic nephropathy
Non-glomerular disease (vascular leakiness)	Acute pyrexial illnesses
	Chronic inflammatory conditions, including obesity and chronic infections
	Smoking
	CVD, especially congestive heart failure

number of inflammatory and vascular conditions (see Table 1.4). Furthermore, it is often transient and reversible. Microalbuminuria is known to increase with age, obesity, and the metabolic syndrome. It is also adversely affected by heavy smoking.

In addition, considerable evidence points to microalbuminuria as a significant CVD risk factor. This is most likely to be due to the known association of microalbuminuria with clinical as well as subclinical manifestations of CVD and the related microinflammatory milieu.

The KDOQI guidelines, which stipulate that microalbuminuria is a marker of CKD, insist on repeated and confirmatory testing with two of three measurements over a 3-month period being abnormal, thus confirming the chronic nature of the microalbuminuria.

Proteinuria/macroalbuminuria

Proteinuria (macroalbuminuria) is a well-known poor prognostic marker in CKD (see Chapter 3). In diabetic nephropathy, it is often associated with progressive diabetic nephropathy. It is also associated with poor CVD outcomes. In non-diabetic CKD, it is generally agreed that proteinuria levels >1g/24h carry a poor prognosis in terms of progression of CKD. In fact, such high levels of proteinuria seem to modulate the impact of systemic hypertension of CKD progression; CKD patients with proteinuria levels <1g/24h appear to have a good prognosis, even in the face of raised blood pressure levels. Conversely, patients with proteinuria >1g/24h have a poor prognosis, even at relatively normal levels of blood pressure. The level of proteinuria may also explain the better outcome of tubulointerstitial nephritis (low proteinuric state) compared to glomerulopathies (high proteinuric state).

Management of proteinuria

Proteinuria in diabetes mellitus

Annual screening for microalbuminuria is recommended as appropriate treatment could reverse and prevent or slow progression to overt diabetic nephropathy. One study suggested that treatment of people with type 2 diabetes with an angiotensin-converting enzyme inhibitor (ACEi) (trandalopril) prevented the onset of microalbuminuria (Ruggenenti, et al., 2004). This awaits confirmation. Treatment of microalbuminuria consists of optimization of diabetes control, control of hypertension, the use of ACEi/angiotensin receptor blocker (ARB) as well as management of dyslipidaemia and cessation of smoking. The reduction of these microalbuminuria-related risk factors has been shown to reduce and, on occasions, reverse microalbuminuria.

Those with macroalbuminuria are at risk of progressive CKD and end-stage renal disease (ESRD) and therefore, should be under close surveillance of kidney function, blood pressure, and CVD risk factors. Treatment with ACEi/ARB is the cornerstone of the management of proteinuric diabetic nephropathy. A number of studies have shown that ACEi, ARB, or a combination of both are effective in controlling hypertension, reducing proteinuria, and slowing the progression of diabetic nephropathy (see Chapter 8). Furthermore, inhibitors of the RAAS, involving renin inhibition (aliskerin) or antagonizing aldosterone such as spironolactone or eplerenone, are also effective at reducing proteinuria in diabetic nephropathy when used in combination with ACEi/ARB.

Caution should be exerted when using inhibitors of the RAAS in diabetic patients with vascular and ischaemic nephropathy as renal function can deteriorate significantly upon the introduction of these antihypertensive agents. Also, recent data from a combination study (ONTARGET) of an ACEi (ramipril) and an ARB (telmisartan) suggest that in patients at high CVD risk, such treatment may compromise renal function and accelerate the decline of kidney function.

Proteinuric CKD

In CKD patients with significant proteinuria (>1g/24h), most guidelines recommend to use ACEi/ARB as initial and preferential antihypertensive agents. This is because ACEi/ARB appear to have the capacity to control hypertension, but also to reduce proteinuria through a number of putative mechanisms, including reduction of intraglomerular hypertension as well as reduction of glomerular permeability to proteins. The NICE UK CKD guidelines recommend ACEi/ARB treatment in nondiabetic and normotensive CKD with proteinuria >1g/24h, although there is little evidence to support such a recommendation.

To optimize the antihypertensive and anti-proteinuric effect of ACEi/ARB, it is recommended to combine such treatment with a reduction in dietary salt and/or diuretic therapy. It has been suggested that whilst treatment should aim to reduce blood pressure to levels <130/80mmHg, it should also be uptitrated to reduce proteinuria to levels <1g/24h. This can also be achieved by a combination of inhibitors of the RAAS.

The inhibition of the RAAS is also the initial treatment of choice to reduce nephrotic range proteinuria in patients with glomerulonephritis and preserved renal function (see 'Practical approach to glomerulonephritis'). In these patients, a significant reduction of proteinuria and improved outcome can be achieved with these agents in the absence of immunosuppression. Also, heavy proteinuria in these patients (>1g/24h) indicates a lower blood pressure target (<125/75mmHg) as with the treatment of patients with overt diabetic nephropathy (see Figure 1.1 and 'Practical approach to diabetic kidney disease').

Proteinuria and pregnancy

Proteinuria in pregnancy can be due to a pregnancy-related disease such as pre-eclampsia or may be a first presentation or worsening of pre-existing CKD. Both pre-eclampsia and CKD are associated with adverse fetal and maternal outcomes and should be referred for specialist input.

Practical approach to haematuria

Microscopic and macroscopic haematuria are health care problems commonly encountered by primary care physicians worldwide. It has

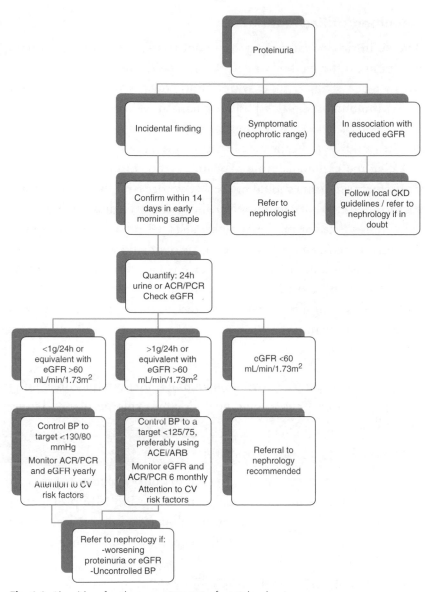

Fig. 1.1 Algorithm for the management of proteinuria

been reported in around 2–9% of the general population. Prevalence reaching as high as 30% has been reported in some developing countries. However, repeated testing has often shown lower values. Around 15% of those presenting with macroscopic haematuria have underlying malignancy.

Definition of haematuria

The definition of microscopic haematuria is debatable and varies according to the method of detection. Significant haematuria refers to any macroscopic/visible, symptomatic microscopic, or persistent, non-symptomatic, dipstick-positive haematuria. Persistent haematuria means two of three positive dipstick tests. Recent dipsticks are highly sensitive and 1+ is diagnostic for haematuria, even if it is haemolyzed (alkaline and hypotonic urine). For microscopic/non-visible diagnosis of haematuria, urine should be freshly voided and this is not always easy to obtain within communities. Microscopic diagnosis of haematuria requires three or more red blood cells per high-power field light microscopy detected in two of three urine sediments from properly collected urine specimens. Haematuria can emanate from the glomeruli or the rest of the urinary tract. Glomerular haematuria is often associated with urine dysmorphic red cells and red cell casts. It is commonly associated with proteinuria >1g/24h.

Causes of haematuria

Causes of haematuria vary from incidental finding to life-threatening urological cancer. Causes could be divided into glomerular and non-glomerular.

Glomerular causes of haematuria

- All forms of glomerulonephritis, primary or secondary, can present with haematuria, usually in association with proteinuria (>1g/24h). Certain forms of glomerulonephritis are characterized by either isolated, persistent, or recurrent bouts of haematuria such as:
  - IgA nephropathy which is one of the most common forms of glomerulonephritis and characterized by recurrent bouts of macroscopic haematuria triggered by associated infections.
- Alport's syndrome: a hereditary condition often associated with hearing defects.
- Benign familial haematuria/thin basement membrane nephropathy.

Non-glomerular causes of haematuria

- Urinary tract infection (UTI).
- Renal calculi.
- Cystic kidney disease, polycystic kidney disease, medullary cystic disease.
- Renal cell carcinoma.
- Urothelial malignancy
- Benign prostatic hypertrophy.
- Prostate cancer.
- Sickle cell disease.
- Crystalluria.
- Renal vein thrombosis.
- Traumatic (catheterization, instrumentation).

Approach to patients with haematuria

Thorough history taking, physical examination, and risk assessment of urothelial cancer are important initial evaluation steps in patients with significant haematuria.

The following should be excluded before further investigations of haematuria.

Other causes of red urine

- Myoglobinuria or haemoglobinuria (both cause false positive dipstick and require microscopy).
- Drug-induced pigmenturia such as rifampicin and doxorubicin.
- Excessive beetroot ingestion.

Transient causes of haematuria

- UTI (dysuria, frequency, flank pain, nitrites, leukocyte esterase, bacteria).
- Menstruation.
- Exercise-induced haematuria.

Haematuria warranting nephrology referral

- When associated with significant proteinuria (>500mg/24h or spot urine protein:creatinine ratio >50mg/mmol).
- Acute or chronic deterioration of kidney function, particularly if the decline is in excess of 4mL/min/year.
- CKD stages 3b, 4, or 5.
- Macroscopic, visible haematuria associated with intercurrent (usually upper respiratory) infection.
- Urine red cell casts or dysmorphic red blood cells.

Haematuria warranting urology referral

- At any age, macroscopic or symptomatic microscopic, non-visible haematuria.
- Non-symptomatic microscopic haematuria ≥40y old.
- Younger patients with high risk of urothelial cancer or abnormal urine cytology (history of smoking, occupational exposure to aromatic amines and benzene dyes as in leather, rubber and tyre industry, or history of urologic neoplasm).

Appropriate investigations of haematuria

- Patients with UTI should be rescreened six weeks after treatment of the infection to confirm resolution of haematuria.
- Imaging of upper urinary tract:
  - Ultrasound is safe, particularly in pregnancy, inexpensive, and can detect solid tumours larger than 3cm.
  - Intravenous urogram (IVU) could identify transitional cell carcinoma more than 3cm in the kidney or ureter.
  - Computed tomography is valuable for renal calculi, small renal, and pararenal abscesses.
- If upper urinary tract imaging does not establish a cause of haematuria, proceed with urine cytology. Positive urine cytology or high-risk patients should be referred to the urologist for cystoscopy to exclude lower urinary tract pathology. Cytology is limited in detecting low grade malignancy or renal cell carcinoma.

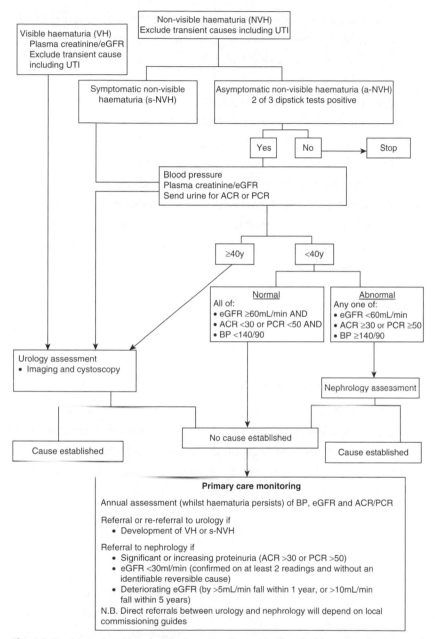

Fig. 1.2 Decision algorithm for the investigation and referral of haematuria. Adapted from UK Renal Association web site: http://www.renal.org/pages/media/Guidelines/RA-BAUS/Haematuria.pdf

- Patients who are suspected of having glomerular haematuria warrant a renal biopsy if it is associated with significant proteinuria (>0.5g/24h) or if it is associated with a significant decline in kidney function (>4/mL/min/y).

- There is no consensus or evidence base for the follow-up of patients with non-identifiable cause for clinically significant haematuria. In one series, it was difficult to reach a diagnosis of 60% of patients with haematuria, whether microscopic or macroscopic. An appropriate approach could be blood pressure check, urine examination and cytology with kidney function assessment every six months. Urine examination is to exclude a new development that warrants a urology or nephrology referral. Yearly cystoscopy for patients ≥40 years or high-risk, young patients (history of smoking, urological malignancy, or occupational exposure to benzene or aromatic amines).

- Figure 1.2 shows the UK Renal Association decision algorithm for the investigation and referral of haematuria.

Practical approach to urinary tract infections (UTIs)

UTIs are common (50–60% of woman will have at least one UTI in their lifetime). UTIs can cause morbidity and mortality in patients with CKD. It is important to distinguish those with CKD who co-incidentally suffer a UTI with no long-term consequences from those who suffer recurrent infections predisposing them to the development of chronic pyelonephritis and CKD. The latter may manifest itself in early childhood and be the presenting feature of an underlying abnormality of the urinary tract that requires urological attention, or be associated with vesicoureteric reflux.

UTI is a common clinical entity that accounts for a significant number of emergency department (ED) or primary care visits. Most patients only require a course of appropriate antibiotics and no further investigations or follow-up. Definitive diagnosis is made by demonstration of bacteriuria (traditionally this is ≥10^5cfu/mL) and leukocytes in the urine. In a proportion of these patients, the diagnosis of UTI may herald the first presentation of CKD.

Where a formal diagnosis of CKD has not been previously established, a clinical history of recurrent UTIs or a complicated UTI may suggest an underlying structural, medical, or neurologic disease. Patients with a neurogenic bladder or bladder diverticulum and post-menopausal women with bladder or uterine prolapse have an increased frequency of UTI due to incomplete bladder emptying. In older men, the incidence of UTI rises because of prostatic obstruction. It is also important to inquire about prior urinary tract manipulation, history of indwelling catheters, or other chronic urinary tract problems because these patients are at much higher risk of UTI. The high urine glucose content and the defective host immune factors in patients with diabetes mellitus also predispose to infection.

Investigations

Most UTIs (even in children) occur in patients with normal urinary tracts and it is important to avoid over-investigation. The identification of bacteriuria is required to confirm a diagnosis of UTI, with a bacterial count of 10^5cfu/mL of urine considered significant. Leukocyturia and nitrites on dipstick provide supportive evidence of infection. Typical causative organisms are shown in Table 1.5.

Further investigation should be considered in patients with:

+ Uncomplicated upper UTI.

+ Complicated UTI (symptomatic infection of any part of the urinary tract, in a patient with functional, metabolic, or structural genitourinary tract abnormalities).

+ Recurrent uncomplicated UTI.

In patients with CKD or known urinary tract structural abnormality, it is important to monitor renal function as this may deteriorate. Imaging studies (a renal ultrasound or dynamic computed tomography (helical CT scan)) should be undertaken if clinical symptoms and signs suggest bladder outlet obstruction or nephrolithiasis. Dynamic CT scans also can serve as a convenient screen in the patient with CKD whose presentation is not typical for UTI, but who has abdominal pain, lower abdominal tenderness, and pyuria.

Table 1.5 Bacterial aetiology of urinary tract infections

Organism	Urinary tract infection (%)	
	Uncomplicated	Complicated
Gram-negative organisms		
Escherichia coli	70–95	21–54
Proteus mirabilis	1–2	1–10
Klebsiella pneumoniae	1–2	2–17
Other	<1	6–20
Gram-positive organisms		
Coagulase-negative *staphylococci*	5–20 or more	1–4
Enterococci	1–2	1–23
Other	<1	2

Management

Antibiotics (guided by likely organism and sensitivities following culture) are the mainstay of treatment for UTI. Adjunctive measures include antipyretics, interventions for the control of pain or nausea, and correction of volume imbalance. Most patients with CKD and uncomplicated CKD may be safely managed at home. Admission should be considered in patients with CKD and an uncomplicated UTI when there are adverse host factors such as age, risk of developing a complicated infection, and likelihood of morbidity associated with failed outpatient treatment.

Generally, patients with complicated UTI should be considered for admission if they have structural abnormalities (e.g. calculi, tract anomalies, indwelling catheter, obstruction) that may affect the response to first-line antibiotics. Similarly patients with CKD who are unable to maintain adequate oral hydration, have minimal home help, and with uncertain compliance with therapy should also be considered for admission. Patients with diabetes and those with recent urinary tract instrumentation, recent hospitalization, or taking broad-spectrum antibiotics have an increased incidence of resistant organisms and, therefore, may need longer therapy.

Urinary tract obstruction

Urinary tract obstruction is an important cause of renal impairment and if left untreated, can lead to irreversible structural damage to the kidney and CKD. Causes of obstruction vary according to age and sex of the patient. Obstruction to the urinary tract should be considered in any patient with unexplained acute (on chronic) or advanced CKD. Investigations to exclude obstruction are mandatory if there are symptoms and signs referrable to the urinary tract (pain, haematuria, lower urinary tract symptoms, distended bladder).

Investigations

Ultrasound scanning (USS) is the most common first-line investigation, although interpretation is operator-dependent. Calyceal dilatation (hydronephrosis) infers obstruction (although non-obstructive urinary tract dilatation may be found in vesicoureteric reflux). The site of the obstruction may be difficult to define on USS. A large distended bladder is diagnostic of bladder outflow obstruction which most commonly occurs as a result of prostatic disease in men. CT and magnetic resonance (MR) scanning are increasingly used to diagnose both the cause and site of obstruction.

Management

Treatment is dictated by the location of the obstruction, the underlying cause, and the degree of renal impairment. Close collaboration between nephrologists, urologists, and radiologists is required. A urinary catheter will effectively relieve bladder outflow obstruction. Upper urinary tract obstruction in the setting of renal impairment may require a nephrostomy as an emergency to allow recovery of renal function whilst definitive surgical treatment is planned. Dialysis should rarely be required, even when there is severe renal impairment.

Following relief of obstruction, there may be a post-obstructive diuresis. Careful and regular assessment of the patient's fluid balance is required with hourly urine volumes and daily serum electrolytes to determine the required rate of fluid and electrolyte replacement; intravenous replacement is commonly required.

Practical approach to hypertension

Hypertension can independently cause CKD, contribute to its development in the setting of other potential kidney diseases, or be the result of CKD. Hypertension is present in over 80% of people with CKD.

The incidence of hypertension increases with worsening CKD. As in patients without kidney disease, the risk of having hypertension in CKD patients is increased with age, higher body mass index (BMI), and in the ethnic minorities.

Hypertension in CKD is, in part, mediated via the RAAS system. Progressive renal insufficiency and subsequent scarring of the kidneys stimulate the release of renin which, through a sequence of steps, leads to secondary hyperaldosteronism, causing salt and water retention. Clinically, the effects are hypertension and volume overload. The RAAS system also leads to vasoconstriction of blood vessels which is further exacerbated by the activation of the sympathetic nervous system. Left ventricular hypertrophy is a well-recognized complication of CKD.

Treatment of renal anaemia with erythropoietin-stimulating agents is thought to aggravate hypertension and patients should have regular monitoring of their blood pressure whilst on treatment.

Progressive CKD leads to hyperphosphataemia, reduced hydroxylation of 25- hydroxycholecalciferol, and secondary hyperparathyroidism. This has been shown to cause hypertension directly and indirectly through the effects of calcium absorption through the gut. Increasing levels of calcium can lead to the deposition within the intimal layer of the arterial wall, causing stiffness and consequent hypertension.

Renovascular disease as a cause of hypertension should be considered when:

- Hypertension remains poorly controlled in compliant patients despite maximum doses of multiple medications.
- There is a significant fall (>25%) in the eGFR following treatment with an ACEi or ARB.
- There is widespread macrovascular disease (arterial bruits).
- There has been flash pulmonary oedema.

Investigation can reveal electrolyte evidence of hyperaldosteronism (hypokalaemia and alkalosis) and asymmetrical kidneys. Renal angiography is the gold standard investigation although MR angiography is frequently used as a screening test. Intervention with renal artery angioplasty and/or stenting may be considered, although the benefit of this on either patient or kidney survival or the ability to control hypertension remains unclear. Before any procedure to the renal arteries, the patient should be counselled about the possibility of acute kidney injury which could be irreversible.

Management

There is strong evidence that effective control of hypertension slows progression of CKD, irrespective of the primary cause. Hypertension is also a strong risk factor for CVD and progressive CKD further increases that risk. Patients with CKD are more likely to succumb to CVD than require renal replacement therapy and therefore, reducing cardiovascular risk, and in particular controlling hypertension, should be the main focus of management.

Proteinuria is now recognized as an independent risk factor for CVD and progressive renal disease in patients with CKD. In patients with proteinuric CKD, hypertension should be treated to a lower target, and ACEis and ARBs should be first-line therapy.

Currently, NICE recommends the following:

- Threshold for treatment as 140/90mmHg.
- Target 120–139/90mmHg.
- Target 120–129/80mmHg if there is proteinuria (ACR >70 or PCR >100mg/mmol).
- ACEi or ARB as first-line agents if ACR >30 or PCR >70mg/mmol.

Patient education is essential to improve concordance with therapy and home monitoring of blood pressure may be helpful.

Non-pharmacological

Weight loss should be encouraged. A drop in 8–10lb (or 4–5kg) can have the same effect as an individual drug and this should be emphasized to patients. Exercise should always be considered as an adjunct to weight loss. The role of excess salt intake as a risk factor for hypertension is controversial, but it is likely that certain populations, such as the elderly, African Americans, and patients with CKD, will benefit from sodium restriction. An alcohol intake above recommended guidelines is a risk factor for hypertension and blood pressure can often be lowered by reducing consumption of alcohol.

Pharmacological

Most patients with CKD will require multiple medications to effectively control their hypertension effectively.

ACEis and ARBs have been shown to slow the progression of kidney disease in patients with diabetes and patients with proteinuric CKD. Concomitantly, they reduce proteinuria. Drugs which interfere with the RAAS system may also reduce mortality in patients with established kidney failure, independent of their effects on blood pressure.

Other classes of medications are frequently required.

- Diuretics are important to control salt and water retention, which may be a key driver for hypertension in CKD. Care must be taken to avoid overdiuresis with hypovolaemia, postural hypotension, and adverse affects on renal function.

- Calcium channel blockers are effective and commonly used in combination with ACEis and ARBs. Their effects on proteinuria are variable, but some studies have shown that they can also reduce proteinuria in patients with CKD.

- Beta-blockers are useful in blocking the alternative mechanism for hypertension—the sympathetic nervous system. These drugs are also cardioprotective and specifically indicated where there is co-existent heart failure.

- Alpha-blockers are a useful adjunct and may help alleviate symptoms of bladder outflow obstruction in men with prostatic disease. However, postural hypotension can occur when high doses are used.

Practical approach to glomerulonephritis

Until recently, chronic glomerulonephrtitis (GN) was the most common cause of ESRD. More recently, diabetic kidney disease and hypertensive nephrosclerosis have become more common. However, acute and chronic GN remain one of the most common nephrological conditions. Whilst most often managed in tertiary referral centres by nephrologists, the early recognition by non-nephrologists of the signs and symptoms of GN allows early referral and effective treatment. Also, increasingly the follow-up of patients affected by chronic GN is devolved to primary care. With that in mind, it is essential that primary care physicians and non-nephrologists have improved insights into the diagnosis and management of GN.

Classification

GN is classified as primary/idiopathic or secondary to infections, vasculitis, neoplasia, toxins, or drugs. It is invariably triggered by an immunological insult: cellular or humoral immunity. This is often manifested by the deposition of immune complexes within the glomerular capillaries and the attraction of inflammatory cells/mediators. Some forms of severe and rapidly progressive GN are due to autoimmunity (against the glomerular basement membrane—Goodpasture's syndrome) and display the deposition in a linear fashion of the autoantibody along the glomerular capillary wall. A third category of glomerular immune injury associated with ANCA-associated systemic vasculitis (AASV) is characterized by a lack (pauci) of immune deposits.

GN is mainly described and classified by the histological type, regardless of the underlying aetiology.

Clinical presentation

GN can present in a number of ways, ranging from mild proteinuria to nephrotic syndrome and/or microscopic haematuria to overt frank haematuria (nephritic syndrome).

Nephrotic syndrome with urinary protein excretion >3.5g/24h is often seen in MCD, FSGS, MN, and MPGN. On the other hand, nephritic syndrome with haematuria, reduced kidney function, hypertension, and oedema is often seen in association with acute GN (post-infectious) (see 'Practical approach to glomerulonephritis') or crescentic/rapidly progressive GN. The latter is characterized by a rapidly declining kidney function, hence the label of rapidly progressive GN.

The prognosis of GN is often a function of the severity and persistence of heavy proteinuria, hypertension as well as the level of renal functional impairment at presentation. All these are poor prognostic factors.

Table 1.6 Description of common forms of GN

Type of GN	Histological description	Electron microscopy	Immunofluorescence
Minimal change disease (MCD)	Normal light microscopy	Effacement of glomerular epithelial (podocytes) foot processes	No deposits
Focal and segmental glomerulosclerosis (FSGS)	Focal (affecting some glomeruli) and segmental (affecting segments of glomeruli) sclerosis/fibrosis of the glomeruli	Small amount of immune deposits can be seen within the glomeruli	IgG and C3 deposits often detected within glomeruli
Mesangioproliferative GN and IgA nephropathy	Proliferation of mesangial cells and expansion of the mesangial matrix	Immune deposits within the mesangium in case of IgA nephropathy	Immune deposits in an arborial distribution within the mesangium, consisting mainly of IgA, IgG, and C3
Membranous nephropathy (MN)	Thickening of the glomerular capillary wall (GBM)	Immune deposits along the subepithelial side of the GBM	IgG, IgM, C3 deposited along the GBM
Membranoproliferative GN (MPGN)	Proliferation of the mesangial cells along with thickneining of the GBM	Immune deposits along the subendothelial side of the GBM (type 1), within the GBM (type 2), and all through the subendothelial, intramembranous, and subepithelial aspects of the GBM (type 3)	IgG, IgM, C3 deposited along the GBM
Crescentic GN	Extraglomerular proliferation of inflammatory cells within the Bowman's space surrounding the glomerular tuft in a crescentic shape	Immune deposits can be seen along the GBM in immune complex-mediated GN, along the GBM in anti-GBM-mediated GN, and scanty immune deposits in AASV (pauci immune deposits)	Three IF patterns can be seen: 1. Granular, immune complex, deposits 2. Linear anti-GBM pattern 3. Pauci immune deposits with fibrin deposits within the Bowman's space

Table 1.7 Clinical features of common forms of GN

Type of GN	Proteinuria	Haematuria	Kidney function	Associations
MCD	+++	+/−	Normal	Most common cause of NS in children
FSGS	++/+++	+	Reduced	African Americans Obesity Recreational drugs HCV HIV
Mesangioproliferative GN and IgA nephropathy (IgAN)	++	++/+++	Normal when isolated haematuria or reduced in IgAN	Primary or secondary to: Alport's syndrome, vasculitides, HSP, SLE. In IgAN, often presenting as recurrent bouts of haematuria associated with intercurrent infections (upper respiratory tract)
MN	+++	++	Reduced	Infections SLE Malignancies Drugs Toxins
Membranoproliferative GN	+++	++	Reduced	HCV infection
Crescentic GN	+/++	+++	Rapidly declining kidney function	Vasculitides: SLE, AASV Anti-GBM disease: Goodpasture's syndrome

Patients with GN presenting with either haematuria, proteinuria, and/or progressively declining kidney function usually undergo a kidney biopsy after the exclusion of other causes of their symptoms and signs. The renal biopsy defines the histological diagnosis as well as the prognosis, based on the severity of the histological, acute inflammatory as well as chronic fibrotic changes. Management is often guided by the severity of these changes.

Referral and management

The management of GN ranges from no intervention and close observations to suppression of proteinuria and/or immunosuppression to control the underlying inflammatory and immune process.

Isolated haematuria is often associated with mild glomerular damage as in mild forms of IgAN, glomerular thin membrane disease, and Alport's syndrome. In the absence of proteinuria and impaired kidney function, isolated haematuria does not warrant treatment. On the other hand, patients with isolated haematuria need to be monitored regularly (annually) for signs of hypertension and decline in kidney function. This should be undertaken in the primary care setting with referral to nephrologists if and when proteinuria (>0.5g/24h) is detected and/or kidney function declines and patients reach CKD stage 3 (eGFR <60mL/min/1.73m^2).

Mild proteinuria (<1g/24h), in the absence of associated haematuria or impaired kidney function (GFR <60mL/min/1.73m^2), should also be managed conservatively in the primary care setting with regular (6-monthly) monitoring. In the presence of either haematuria or impaired kidney function, the patient should be referred to a nephrologist for further investigation and management advice.

Moderate proteinuria (>1g/24h) should be referred to a nephrologist for further investigation. It also warrants treatment with an inhibitor of the RAAS as it is often associated with poor prognosis and decline in kidney function. Management of proteinuria consists of ACEi/ARB, low salt diet, and diuretic therapy as well as the consideration of combining an ACEi and ARB. Blood pressure control aims for target levels <130/80mmHg.

In patients with MCD, steroid therapy is recommended as it induces remission in the majority of patients within four to eight weeks. Patients should be treated with steroids (prednisolone) orally at a starting dose of 1mg/kg/day (~60mg/day in adults) for an initial period of four weeks. The dose should be tapered subsequently. In FSGS, recommendations are of a more prolonged high dose (prednisolone: 60mg/day for eight weeks) to induce remission and avoid frequent relapses. In both conditions, fast tapering of steroids dosage can lead to early and frequent relapses.

In patients with MCD who are either steroid-resistant or steroid-dependent, combination with an alkylating agent such as cyclophosphamide (1–2mg/kg/day) for an 8-week period is known to induce sustained remission.

For steroid-resistant patients with FSGS, combination therapy with cyclosporin (2–3mg/kg/day) has been advocated for a period of 18–24 months.

In patients with progressive MN, heavy proteinuria (>3–5g/24h), and declining kidney function, steroids alone have been found to be ineffective. Consequently, a number of regimen has been advocated, combining steroids with cyclophosphamide, chlorambucil, cyclosporine, or azathioprine. Some have advocated the use of mycophenolate mofetil. More recently, some have suggested that B cell depletion with an anti-CD20 monoclonal antibody (rituximab) was effective at inducing remission in refractory cases. Most of these observations are based on a limited number of cases and await confirmation by large-scale, randomized control clinical trials (RCTs).

Patients with rapidly progressive GN, whether it is idiopathic or secondary to an underlying vasculitis, should be treated early and aggressively with a combination of immunosuppressive agents, including steroids and cyclophosphamide, and occasionally, plasma exchange in those with Goodpasture's syndrome, lung haemorrhage as well as patients with AASV and advanced renal insufficiency (serum creatinine >600umol/L or those who are dialysis-dependent). Combination therapy with steroids and pulse intravenous cyclophosphamide has also been advocated for the management of severe lupus nephritis. In these conditions, it is important that treatment is undertaken in specialized centres with experience in the management of immunosuppression and its complications.

Conclusion

GN is a common nephrological condition. It warrants early detection and intervention. These range from close monitoring, ACE inhibition to control the associated proteinuria and prevent progression to immunosuppression to control the underlying immune-mediated inflammatory process.

Practical approach to diabetic kidney disease

Epidemiology

Worldwide, there is a steady increase in the number of people suffering from diabetes mellitus (DM). It is estimated that by 2030, the global number of people with DM will exceed 350 million. The increase will affect predominantly emerging economies where the prevalence of DM is expected to treble from 2010 to 2030. This global increase is, to a large extent, attributable to an increase in type 2 DM linked to urbanization and the associated obesity—diabesity.

The increase in the number of people with DM and, in particular type 2 DM, has impacted on the number of people suffering from CKD worldwide. DM and hypertension are the two main causes of CKD worldwide and constitute the majority of patients requiring renal replacement therapy (RRT). In fact, in the United States (US), around 40% of all those treated by dialysis are diabetics. In the UK, the prevalence of diabetic nephropathy (DN) amongst patients starting RRT is reaching 20%. Therefore, it is imperative to have a good understanding of the risk factors associated with the development of DM as well as its macrovascular and microvascular complications.

Causes

DM can affect the kidneys through a number of pathways (Table 1.8). Essentially, the kidneys can be involved through microvascular disease affecting the glomeruli and causing the typical DN associated with

Table 1.8 Major causes of kidney disease in people with diabetes

Type of diabetic kidney disease	Manifestation
DN	Affects ~20–40% of type 1 DM. Progressive increase in proteinuria, reaching nephrotic range associated with a decline in kidney function. 20% reach ESRD.
Diabetic renal vascular disease (DRVD)	Affects ~30–50% of type 2 DM. Often preceded and associated with systemic hypertension and diffuse atherosclerosis. Minimal proteinuria and slow renal functional decline.
Bladder autonomic dysfunction	Associated with obstructive uropathy and recurrent UTIs.
Recurrent UTIs	The diabetic milieu, glycosuria, and bladder dysfunction predispose to recurrent UTIs.
Papillary necrosis	The combination of renal ischaemia/hypoxia as well as hyperglycaemic hyperosmolarity leads to renal papillary necrosis, presenting as recurrent bouts of renal colics.
Nephrotoxicity	DKD is susceptible to bouts of acute on CKD due to the nephrotoxicity of radiocontrast material as well as that of drugs such as NSAIDs.
Infections	Besides recurrent UTIs, the diabetic kidney is also susceptible to acute on CKD due to systemic infections, including cutaneous streptococcal infections associated with post-infections proliferative glomerulonephritis.

glomerular hyalinosis and sclerosis described by Kimmelstiel and Wilson. The kidney can also be affected as part of the generalized diffuse atherosclerosis characteristic of diabetic macrovascular complication, leading to atherosclerotic renal vascular disease (ARVD) and ischaemic nephropathy. Clearly, changes associated with diabetic microvascular and macrovascular disease can simultaneously affect the kidney.

Ischaemic nephropathy often affects the renal medulla, which is most susceptible to renal ischaemia and hypoxia, causing papillary necrosis with occasional sloughing of necrotic papilla and simulating renal colics.

Also, people with DM are known to be at risk of autonomic nervous system dysfunction, affecting the bladder and leading to poor voiding and associated recurrent UTIs and obstructive uropathy.

People with DM and DN are at increased risk of nephrotoxicity, including that associated with radiocontrast material used in imaging, but also drug-induced nephrotoxicity, including that associated with non-steroidal anti-inflammatory drugs (NSAIDs). In that respect, people with diabetic vascular nephropathy are also at increased risk of nephrotoxicity due to inhibitors of the RAAS system.

Therefore, it is imperative to bear the range of diabetic kidney complications in mind when dealing with a patient with DM and renal involvement. All too often, diabetic kidney disease equates exclusively with DN, thus limiting the therapeutic scope and also risking mismanagement.

Risk factors

The risk factors associated with the development of DN in patients with type 1 DM include modifiable and non-modifiable risks as listed in Table 1.9. Control of modifiable risk factors can attenuate the development of DN.

Regarding the risk factors associated with DRVD, these are likely to be common to those implicated in the development of atherosclerosis, including age, hypertension, hyperlipidaemia, obesity, and smoking.

Table 1.9 Risk factors associated with the onset of DN

Non-modifiable	Modifiable
Genetic	Glycaemia
Familial	Blood pressure
Race and ethnicity	Dyslipidaemia
	Smoking

Presentation and natural history

Diabetic nephropathy (DN)

DN is a manifestation of diabetic microvascular complications affecting the glomerular capillaries. It is often associated with a parallel development of other microvascular complications such as retinopathy and neuropathy.

Whether it affects type 1 or type 2 DM, the onset of DN is likely to take place a few years (5–8) after the onset of DM. Whilst this is easily determined in type 1, insulin-dependent DM, it is more difficult to determine in type 2 DM as the onset of the disease often goes unrecognized for many years.

The onset of DN is characterized by the appearance of microalbuminuria (MA) (urine albumin excretion rate between 30 and 300mg/24h and below standard dipstick test detection level (see Table 1.1). The onset of MA is influenced by the factors listed above, including the quality of glycaemia control, blood pressure level, hyperlipidaemia as well as smoking during the first years following the diagnosis of DM. MA affects about 20–40% of people with DM. Although high level MA progresses after a few years to overt proteinuria and DN, MA has the potential to be reversible if a number of risk factors are corrected in time. As will be discussed below, it can also be reduced by the inhibition of the RAAS.

MA will progress in some patients to overt proteinuria/albuminuria detectable by dipstick testing (>300mg/24h). The progression of overt diabetic is associated with the steady decline in renal function, from glomerular hyperfiltration (during the stage of latent nephropathy and MA) to CKD stage 3 (eGFR <60mL/min/1.73m²). With time, increasing levels of proteinuria/albuminuria will be associated with declining renal function until it reaches ESRD when the GFR is less than 15mL/min. Progression from MA to ESRD (CKD stage 5) takes, on average, 10–15 years as the average annual rate of decline of GFR is around 5mL/min/year in DN.

It is important to appreciate that DN is often (up to 60%) associated with microscopic haematuria.

Table 1.10 Factors affecting the progression of DN

Non-modifiable	Modifiable
Genetic	Hypertension
Familial	Proteinuria
Race and ethnicity	Hyperglycaemia
	Dyslipidaemia
	Smoking

The course of DN in type 1 and 2 DM is comparable. Ultimately, around 20% of patients with DM will reach ESRD unless they succumb during CKD stage 3 or 4 to their cardiovascular complications.

Diabetic renal vascular disease (DRVD)

DRVD is an integral part of diabetic macrovascular atherosclerotic complications, causing coronary artery, cerebrovascular and peripheral vascular diseases. Patients often give a history of long-standing hypertension and related CVD complications.

This type of DKD can be distinguished from DN by the low level of proteinuria (<1g/24h), refractory systolic hypertension as well as the variable rate of kidney function decline. Microscopic haematuria can also be a feature of DRVD. Control of systemic hypertension and reduction of the CVD risks can favourably affect the outcome. Patients with severe and diffuse, diabetic, macrovascular complications are at increased risk of CVD morbidity and mortality.

Cardiovascular complications in DM are affected by renal involvement. Overall and CVD death are proportional to the severity of albuminuria/ proteinuria. Also, a reduction of kidney function is associated with increased CVD mortality. Therefore, CVD complications in DM are the result of the triple hit of hyperglycaemia, hypertension, and CKD.

It is important to recognize that a number of people with DM (up to 30% according to some series), especially those suffering from type 2 DM, have unrelated glomerulonephritis such as membranous or membranoproliferative nephropathies. Those are characterized by the sudden onset of heavy proteinuria and/or haematuria in the absence of a history of gradual decline in renal function or in the absence of a detectable association with microvascular or macrovascular disease. In such instance, a renal biopsy is indicated to elucidate the nature of the renal pathology and guide management.

Management

Microalbuminuria (MA)

Early detection of MA is essential for prompt management and improved outcome. Most national and international guidelines stipulate that people with DM should be screened annually for MA.

Once detected, a concerted effort should be made to reverse all the associated predisposing factors such as poor DM control, raised blood pressure level, dyslipidaemia, and smoking. The cornerstone of the management of MA is the optimization of DM control. The chance of reversibility of MA to normoalbuminuria depends on the correction of as many risk factors as possible: hyperglycaemia, hypertension, hyperlipidaemia, and cessation of smoking. Also, MA is often associated with elevated blood pressure levels and therefore, warrants prompt initiation of antihypertensive therapy with an inhibitor of the RAAS. Consequently, a number of reports show reversal of MA and improved renal and CVD outcomes.

Overt DN

Control of hypertension Established DN is often associated with poor glycaemia control as well as hypertension. For that, the cornerstone of the management of established and overt DN is the control of hypertension. Most guidelines (reviewed in Chapter 8) recommend the use of inhibitors of the RAAS such as ACEis or ARBs as first-line treatment. They also recommend lower target blood pressure levels than those recommended for non-diabetic, non-proteinuric CKD (<125/75mmHg).

A number of analyses and studies such as the UK Prospective Diabetes Study (UKPDS) and the Appropriate Blood Pressure Control in Diabetes (ABCD) study suggests that the lower the blood pressure, the better the outcome of microvascular disease in DM, including DN.

This often requires more than one antihypertensive agent, starting with an ACEi/ARB, then combination with a diuretic to optimize the effect of the ACEi/ARB, then the addition of other agents as indicated, including beta-blockers for cardioprotection and calcium antagonists. The choice of the antihypertensive agent for the treatment of overt DN is also guided by the anti-proteinuric effect of the agent, ACEi/ARB being the most anti-proteinuric agents whilst diuretics have the advantage of a synergistic antihypertensive and anti-proteinuric effect with inhibitors of the RAAS. The anti-proteinuric effects of ACEi/ARB has been attributed to the control of systemic hypertension, but also to a reduction of intraglomerular hypertension as well as glomerular

permeability to proteins. Other agents with anti-proteinuric pro-
perties are the non-dihydropyridine calcium antagonists (diltiazem
and verapamil) whilst beta-blockers having little anti-proteinuric
effect.

In order to maximize the anti-proteinuric effect of the management
of DN (target levels <1g/24h), combination therapy including an ACEi
and ARB has been recommended. Also, combination therapy including
a renin inhibitor (aliskerin) and an ARB has been shown to be effective.
However, caution should be exerted when initiating such combinations
as a recent report suggested worsening renal outcomes in patients at
high CVD risk, including diabetics with such therapy (ONTARGET
clinical trial).

Finally, it has been suggested that inhibitors of the RAAS have cardioprotective effects in patients with DN. They have been shown to reduce
morbidity and mortality. However, debate continues as to whether
such cardioprotection is independent of a better blood pressure control
compared to other agents.

A word of caution is warranted regarding the use of RAAS inhibitors
in CKD, including DN. These agents can be associated with a significant reduction in kidney function. Therefore, it is advisable to closely
monitor (within a week from initiation or changes of dosage) renal
function (serum creatinine and eGFR). A fall in eGFR by more that
20% warrants further monitoring (at four weeks) whilst a fall by 25%
or more warrants the discontinuation of therapy.

Also, caution should be exerted in the prescription of these agents to
patients with DRVD as they can cause a serious deterioration in kidney
function and even precipitate ESRD. In the absence of typical DN with
proteinuria >1g/24h, these agents should not be used.

Control of glycaemia A number of observations and studies such as
DCCT and UKPDS have suggested that control of DM and glycaemia
(target HbA1c ~7%) has a beneficial effect on diabetic complications,
including nephropathy. However, recent data from ACCORD and
ADVANCE studies have raised some reservations regarding overzeal-
ous reduction of glycaemia as the former showed worsening CVD outcomes whilst the latter failed to show an advantage.

Other interventions Correction of dyslipidaemia and cessation of smoking are also key components of the management of DN. These interventions also have the added advantage of reducing CVD risk. This is a very important goal of the management of patients with diabetic kidney disease as CVD constitute the major cause of morbidity and mortality.

Intensive multifactorial intervention It is important to appreciate that the ultimate goal of reducing the complications of DM, including DKD and CVD, depends on a multifactorial approach relying of maximizing glycaemia control (HbA1c ~7%), reducing blood pressure (<125/75mmHg), the use of a statin to reduce hypercholesterolaemia as well as cessation of smoking. Such a multifactorial aggressive approach has been shown by the Steno group in Denmark to yield better macrovascular and microvascular outcomes when compared to standard therapies.

Table 1.11 Interventions to slow the progression of DN

Intervention	Target
Blood pressure control	<125/75mmHg
Proteinuria reduction	<1g/24h; PCR <100mg/mmol
Glycaemia control	HbA1c ~7%
Dyslipidaemia control	Total cholesterol <5mmol/L
	LDL cholesterol <2mmol/L
Smoking	Cessation
Dietary protein intake	~0.8g/kg/day

Conclusion

DN is preventable, detectable, and treatable.

Practical approach to drugs in CKD

Medicines management in any chronic disease is crucial. This may be particularly challenging in CKD because of the difficulties associated with prescribing in patients with reduced renal function. Once a diagnosis of CKD has been established, it is essential that the potential effects of any therapeutic intervention on the kidney are considered. Dosing of any drug which relies on a renal route of excretion needs to be adjusted appropriately to avoid accumulation of the parent drug and its metabolites with ensuing potential toxicity. This is a particular problem in the elderly who frequently have impaired renal function and commonly have a low functional renal reserve. In addition, pharmacokinetic changes may markedly increase tissue drug concentrations during acute illnesses as a result of a rapid reduction in renal clearance, especially if accompanied by dehydration. Medicines that are safe in health can suddenly become nephrotoxic. For these reasons, those drugs with a narrow therapeutic window or a known predictable adverse effects on renal function should generally be avoided when renal function is poor. For example, a patient stabilized on a drug with a narrow margin between the therapeutic and the toxic dose (e.g. digoxin) can rapidly develop adverse effects in the aftermath of a myocardial infarction or a respiratory tract infection.

The prevalence of CKD increases with age as does the incidence of comorbidity. Patients with multiple diseases are likely to be prescribed a number of medications (polypharmacy) and may be particularly susceptible to the reduced renal clearance in CKD, predisposing to vague and non-specific adverse reactions. Confusion, constipation, bleeding, and postural hypotension are frequently reported by those on antihypertensive, diuretic, or non-steroidal anti-inflammatory medications. Finally, some drugs are not effective when patients have CKD, limiting therapeutic options and increasing morbidity.

Diuretics

Diuretics are commonly prescribed to treat salt and water excess in patients with CKD and should be reviewed on a regular basis. Overdiuresis should be avoided since this will adversely affect renal perfusion and function, and cause postural hypotension. The lowest effective dose to stimulate the required diuresis and maintain euvolaemia should be prescribed. In patients with CKD, larger doses may be needed to compensate for the reduced filtration rate.

NSAIDs

Bleeding associated with aspirin and other NSAIDs is more common in patients with CKD and are more likely to have a fatal or serious outcome. Such drugs should be used with caution in CKD since uraemia per se causes platelet dysfunction, predisposing to spontaneous bleeding especially in the elderly. NSAIDs predictably reduce GFR and may cause salt and water retention, worsening the control of hypertension. They may pose a special hazard in the elderly and patients with cardiac disease, both of whom are likely to have co-existing CKD.

Other drugs

Other drugs which commonly cause adverse reactions are antihypertensives, metformin, digoxin, and those which are excreted through the kidneys, but have long half-lives. ACEis and ARBs may result in an unacceptable fall in renal function, especially in patients with renal artery stenosis, and if it occurs, it should prompt further investigation for this condition. The use of metformin should be reviewed in any patient whose eGFR falls $<45mL/min/1.73m^2$ and should be discontinued once the eGFR is $<30mL/min/1.73m^2$. The usual maintenance dose of digoxin in patients with CKD is 62.5µg daily and higher does may result in toxicity.

Doses

Before prescribing any drug, it is prudent to consult an approved for mulary (e.g. British National Formulary (BNF)) and verify the correct dose appropriate for the degree of CKD. Unfortunately, many formularies use vague terms such as 'reduce the dose in mild or moderate renal impairment', which can be unhelpful to the clinician and leads to an inconsistent approach. Serum creatinine may be used to assess renal function, but this may not accurately reflect the kidney function of an individual since its level also depends on muscle mass (and hence, age, sex, and race). In particular, elderly females may have significant impairment of renal function despite a normal or near normal serum creatinine. Renal function is more commonly (universally within the UK) expressed as an estimated GFR (eGFR) which is calculated from the Modification of Diet in Renal Disease (MDRD) study formula that uses serum creatinine, age, sex, and race. This offers an opportunity to provide consistent advice about the appropriate dose adjustment and avoidance of potentially toxic drugs at various stages of CKD, but has not yet been widely adopted by formularies.

Generally, prescribing should be kept to a minimum in all patients with severe CKD. With earlier stages of CKD, renal function should be checked before prescribing any drug and appropriate dose modification made. Many antibiotics require dose adjustment (reduction) when renal function is impaired.

In patients who have CKD stage 5 or who are on RRT, it is good practice to liaise with specialists (e.g. renal pharmacists, specialist nurses, dieticians, or clinicians) in regard to changes with medications.

References

Ahmed, A., El-Nahas, A.M., 2009. Management of hypertension in chronic kidney disease. In: Molony, D.A., Craig, J.C., eds. *Evidence-based nephrology*. Wiley–Blackwell, pp.214–22.

Barit, D., Cooper, M.E., 2008. Diabetic patients and kidney protection: an attainable target. *Journal of Hypertension*, 26(Suppl 2), S3–7.

Cattran, D., 2005. Management of membranous nephropathy: when and what for treatment. *Journal of the American Society of Nephrology*, 16(5), pp.1188–94.

de Jong, P.E., Gansevoort, R.T., 2009. Focus on microalbuminuria to improve cardiac and renal protection. *Nephron Clinical Practice*, 111(3), c204–10.

Harris, K.P.G., 2006. Urinary tract obstruction. In: Johnson, R., Feehally, J., Floege, J., eds. *Comprehensive clinical nephrology*. 3rd ed. Mosby, pp. 657–70.

Klinger, M., Mazanowska, O., 2008. Primary idiopathic glomerulonephritis: modern algorithm for diagnosis and treatment. *Polskie Archiwum Medycyny Wewnetrznel*, 118(10), pp.567–71.

McDonald, M.M., Swagerty, D., Wetzel, L., 2006. Assessment of microscopic haematuria in adults. *American Family Physician Journal*, 73(10), pp.1748–54. http://www.renal.org/pages/media/Guidelines/RA-BAUS/Haematuria.pdf.

National Institute for Health and Clinical Excellence, 2008. Chronic kidney disease: national clinical guideline for early identification and management in adults in primary and secondary care. NICE: CG73. London: The Royal College of Physicians. Available at: http://www.nice.org.uk/nicemedia/pdf/CG073FullGuideline.pdf

Radbill, B., Murphy, B., LeRoith, D., 2008. Rationale and strategies for early detection and management of diabetic kidney disease. *Mayo Clinical Proceedings*, 83(12), pp.1373–81.

Ruggenenti, P., Fassi, A., Ilieva, A.P., Bruno, S., Iliev, I.P., Brusegan, V., Rubis, N., Gherardi, G., Arnoldi, F., Ganeva, M., Ena-lordache, B., Gaspari, F., Perna, A., Bossi, A., Trevisan, R., Dodesini, A.R., Remuzzi, G., 2004. Bergamo Nephrologic Diabetes Complications Trial (BENEDICT) Investigators. Preventing microalbu- minuria in type 2 diabetes. *The New England Journal of Medicine*, 351(19), pp. 1941–51. Epub 2004 Oct 31.

Schernthaner, G., 2009. Kidney disease in diabetology: lessons from 2008. *Nephrology Dialysis Transplantion*, 24(2), pp.396–9.

Schollum, J., 2009. Upper and lower urinary tract infection in adults. In: Barratt, E.J., Harris, K., Topham, P., eds. *Oxford desk reference of nephrology*. Oxford: Oxford University Press.

Troyanov, S., Wall, C.A., Miller, J.A., Scholey, J.W., Cattran, D.C.; Toronto Glomerulonephritis Registry Group, 2005. Focal and segmental glomerulosclero- sis: definition and relevance of a partial remission. *Journal of the American Society of Nephrology*, 16(4), pp.1061–8.

van der Velde, M., Halbesma, N., de Charro, F.T., Bakker, S.J., de Zeeuw, D., de Jong, P.E., Gansevoort, R.T. 2009. Screening for albuminuria identifies individuals at increased renal risk. *Journal of the American Society of Nephrology*, 20(4), pp.852–62.

Chapter 2

Chronic kidney disease (CKD): the scope of the global problem

Anne T. Reutens and Robert C. Atkins

Definition of chronic kidney disease (CKD) according to the National Kidney Foundation (NKF) and Kidney Disease: Improving Global Outcomes (KDIGO)

* Structural or functional abnormalities of the kidneys for ≥3 months, manifested by:
  * Either kidney damage (pathologic abnormalities, markers of renal damage in urine or blood, or imaging abnormalities).
  * Or GFR <60mL/min/1.73m^2 (with or without kidney damage) (Levey, et al., 2005; Levey, et al., 2007a).

Classification of CKD as defined by KDOQI and modified and endorsed by KDIGO

This is the currently preferred staging and classification system for use in epidemiologic studies for estimating the global burden of CKD.

Table 2.1 Staging of CKD

Stage	Description	GFR (mL/min/1.73m^2)
1	Kidney damage with normal or increased GFR	≥90
2	Kidney damage with mild decreased GFR	60–89
3	Moderately decreased GFR	30–59
4	Severely decreased GFR	15–29
5	Kidney failure	<15 (or dialysis)

TREATMENT stages 1–5: T=kidney transplant recipient; stage 5: D=dialysis recipient

* Estimated GFR (eGFR) is calculated from serum creatinine by equations such as the modified four-variable Modification of Diet in

Renal Disease (MDRD) study equation (Levey, et al., 1999; Levey, et al., 2007b). Another equation that is used to derive eGFR from serum creatinine is the Cockcroft–Gault (CG) equation.

◆ Potential problems with this classification are discussed in a recent mini-review (Glassock & Winearls, 2008). In summary, these problems include:

• The inaccuracy of eGFR when compared to direct GFR measurement in the eGFR range $> 60mL/min/1.73$ m^2.

• The validity of using the unmodified MDRD equation to estimate GFR in populations that differ in ethnicity from the population of the original study that was used to derive the equation.

• Questions on the use of microalbuminuria to define CKD stage 1 in some non-diabetic people such as obese individuals in whom microalbuminuria is common.

• The debate on whether the healthy elderly who have a decreased eGFR should be classified as having CKD without regards to age-specific eGFR ranges.

◆ Therefore, there may be inherent overestimation of CKD burden when this classification is used.

Use of the NKF-KDIGO classification in population estimates of CKD prevalence

◆ To estimate CKD prevalence, representative, randomized, cross-sectional, population-wide sampling is required to make valid inferences on the prevalence in the target population. Examples of well-conducted population-wide surveys include the National Health and Nutrition Examination Survey (NHANES) in the US (available at: http://www.cdc.gov/nchs/about/major/nhanes/datalink.htm) and the AusDiab study in Australia (Atkins, et al., 2004; Barr, et al., 2005).

◆ The adequacy of the sampling design, i.e. whether it is a truly unbiased sample, must be considered when interpreting the results. For example, estimates of CKD prevalence from a referred population such as those attending medical clinics overestimate the prevalence;

NHANES was a survey of households, so only included adults who were civilians (not including military personnel) and non-institutionalized (not inclusive of prisoners or elderly residents in nursing homes, a population in which a high prevalence of CKD is likely).

♦ These cross-sectional population-wide surveys often have one study visit for the participant, so it is impossible to verify the persistence of the condition (i.e. to fulfil the 3-month criterion of the KDIGO classification). This can lead to overestimation of the prevalence.

♦ Some population surveys examined the urine only for microalbuminuria. Other urine indicators of renal damage e.g. haematuria, were not included. This may lead to an underestimate of the prevalence of the earlier CKD stages (1 and 2).

Definition of end-stage renal disease (ESRD)

Chronic kidney disease where kidney function is reduced to the extent that renal replacement therapy (RRT), i.e. dialysis or kidney transplant, is required to sustain life.

Note that CKD stage 5 and ESRD are not synonymous because:

♦ Not all people with GFR $<15\text{mL/min}/1.73\text{m}^2$ receive RRT.

♦ Some symptomatic people with GFR $>15\text{mL/min}/1.73\text{m}^2$ may receive RRT.

♦ Kidney transplant recipients often have GFRs $>15\text{mL/min}/1.73\text{m}^2$.

Problems with international comparisons of ESRD data

♦ ESRD data are derived from national renal registries of RRT patients.

♦ Some registries have >90% coverage of all RRT patients within the country, either because of compulsory reporting (US) or good voluntary reporting systems (Australia and New Zealand, Japan, Canada). Data from countries in which the voluntary submission of information to the registries of ESRD data is lower will underestimate ESRD prevalence (Schena, 2000).

♦ Because access to RRT depends on the local health care system, renal registries in countries with low access will underestimate ESRD prevalence because people die before receiving RRT as they cannot afford RRT or the availability of RRT is severely restricted. RRT access reflects the national gross domestic product (Schena, 2000).

• National renal registries do not have a uniform reporting system. The US Renal Data System (USRDS) reports only people who have survived to day 90 (i.e. it excludes those who died soon after starting RRT) (USRDS, 2007), while other registries report patients from day 1 of RRT.

• Therefore, in this chapter, renal registry data are referred to as 'treated ESRD' data to reflect the fact that these are probably underestimates of the true ESRD prevalence.

Prevalence of CKD in Western countries

International comparisons of CKD prevalence have been reviewed previously (Glassock & Winearls, 2008; Zhang & Rothenbacher, 2008).

US

Age-adjusted CKD prevalence estimates for stages 1–4 were obtained from NHANES 1988–1994 and 1999–2006 (Coresh, et al., 2007; USRDS, 2008).

• The prevalence of impaired GFR ($<60mL/min/1.73m^2$) increased from 5.7% in 1988–1994 to 8.1% in 2003–2006.

• Impaired GFR was more common in adults ≥60 years of age (0.6% at age 20–39 years; 4.4% at age 40–59 years; 28.1% at age 60 years or older in 2003–2006).

• Impaired GFR was more common in diabetics.

• The prevalence of albuminuria was relatively stable (8.7% in 1988–1994; 9.3% in 2003–2006).

• Albuminuria was most prevalent in those aged ≥60 years, African Americans, people with hypertension, and those with diabetes.

• The prevalence of the composite disorder of impaired GFR or microalbuminuria increased from 12.4% in 1988–1994 to 15.0% in 2003–2006.

• The prevalence of the composite disorder was high in those aged 60 years or older (37.8% in 2003–2006).

Table 2.2 Estimated prevalence of CKD in Western countries, derived from population-based surveys

Country	Study	Reference	Study design, number of participants (n), age group, comments	Prevalence of CKD stage (%)							
				1–5	3–5	1–4	1	2	3	4	5
US	NHANES 1999–2006	USRDS, 2008	Nationally representative, cross-sectional, continuous survey of the civilian non-institutionalized population aged ≥20 years, (n = 18, 212).	15.0**	8.1**	NR	3.2 (4.6)*	4.1 (6.0)*	7.8	0.5 (stages 4–5)	NR
US	NHANES 1999–2004	Coresh, et al., 2007	As above, n=13, 233.	NR	NR	13.1 (11.1 male; 15.0 female)	1.8	3.2	7.7	0.35	NR
Norway	HUNT II	Hallan, et al., 2006	Population-based health survey of Nord-Trøndelag County of adults ≥20 years from 1995–1997. The county was representative of the general Norwegian population and the participation rate was 70.4%. Study participants were 97% white, n=65,181.	NR	NR	10.2	2.7*	3.2*	4.2	0.2	NR

(Continued)

Table 2.2 (Continued) Estimated prevalence of CKD in Western countries, derived from population-based surveys

Country	Study	Reference	Study design, number of participants (n), age group, comments	Prevalence of CKD stage (%)							
				1–5	3–5	1–4	1	2	3	4	5
Iceland	Reykjavik Heart Study	Viktorsdottir, et al., 2005	Population-based cohort study of adults resident in Reykjavik in 1967 born in 1907–1935. Participation rate was ~70%, age 33–85 years, n=19,256, all were white.	12.5 (female); 7 (male)	11.6 (female); 4.7 (male)	NR	0.9 (female); 2.4 (male) (stages 1–2)	NR		NR	NR
Netherlands	PREVEND (Prevention of Renal and Vascular End Stage Disease)	de Zeeuw, et al., 2005; Gansevoort, et al., 2005; Verhave, et al., 2005	Residents of Groningen aged 28–75 years were invited to participate. The participation rate was 10% (n=8,592). The prevalence of risk factors in the participants was comparable to national prevalence. The original sample was enriched for the presence of micro-albuminuria.	17.6 (10.4)	NR	NR	2.7 (1.3)	9.1 (3.8)	5.7 (5.3)	0.15 (0.04)	0.04 (0)

Table 2.2 (Continued) Estimated prevalence of CKD in Western countries, derived from population-based surveys

Country	Study	Reference	Study design, number of participants (n), age group, comments	Prevalence of CKD stage (%)							
				1–5	3–5	1–4	1	2	3	4	5
			Adjustment was made to the prevalence of CKD stages, based on a subsequent truly random sample of the population (n=2,489) (de Zeeuw, et al., 2005) and these adjusted figures are shown in this table in brackets.								
Italy	Gubbio population study	Cirillo, et al., 2006	Population-based cohort study of adults resident in the central Italian town of Gubbio, n=4,574, aged 18–95 years.	NR	6.2 (female); 5.7 (male)	NR	NR	NR	NR	NR	NR
Spain	EPIRCE (Studio Epidemio- lógico de la Insuficiencia Renal en España)	Otero, et al., 2005	Spanish general population-based, cross-sectional study of randomly selected adults ≥20 years. Pilot study analysis limited to the residents of the region of Galicia, n=237, small sample size.	12.7	NR	NR	3.5	3.5	5.3	0.4	0

(Continued)

Table 2.2 (Continued) Estimated prevalence of CKD in Western countries, derived from population-based surveys

Country	Study	Reference	Study design, number of participants (n), age group, comments	Prevalence of CKD stage (%)							
				1–5	3–5	1–4	1	2	3	4	5
Switzerland	SAPALDIA 2	Nitsch, et al., 2006	Cross-sectional random sample of the Swiss population, n=6,317. The nitial study was in 1991 and the follow-up study was in 2002–2003. No microalbuminuria data.	NR	Age <55 yrs: 1.1 (male), 7.9 (female) Age 55–65 years: 7.1 (male, 23.5 female) Age >65 years: 12.9 male, 35.9 female	NR	NR	NR	NR	NR	NR
Austra ia	AusDiab	Polkinghorne, et al., 2008	National baseline survey conducted in 1999–2000 of the general Australia population aged ≥25 years, n=11,247.	13.4	7.7	12.1	1.4	4.3	7.5	0.28	0.01

NR=not reported; * Gender-specific microalbuminuria criteria; ** 2003–2006

To determine any change in CKD risk factors over time, the prevalence of cigarette smoking, obesity, hypertension, high cholesterol, and diabetes in adults with either CKD stage 3 or albuminuria were compared using data from NHANES 1988–1994 and 1999–2004 (Fox & Muntner, 2008).

- Statistically significant falls in prevalence ratios for obesity, hypertension, and high cholesterol were found, suggesting that the management of these factors had improved.

- There were no changes in the prevalence ratios for diabetes or for smoking.

Europe

The Norwegian HUNT II study (Hallan, et al., 2006a) was one of the few in which the study protocol was designed to confirm the persistence of microalbuminuria. Three urine samples were obtained and the persistence of microalbuminuria was defined as two or three abnormal ACR measurements.

Australia

The overall prevalence of CKD stages 1–5 in the AusDiab study was analyzed using creatinine assays calibrated with isotope dilution mass spectrometry. The eGFR was calculated using the MDRD formula, in conjunction with urinalysis results (Polkinghorne, et al., 2008).

- The prevalence of impaired GFR (<60mL/min/1.73m^2) was 7.7% (5.9% of males and 9.4% of females).

- The prevalence of impaired GFR increased significantly with age; in those <65 years, the prevalence was 2.4% and in those ≥65 years, the prevalence was 30.4%.

- Impaired GFR was present in 18.4% of those with diabetes and 18.0% of those with hypertension.

- Microalbuminuria was present in 6.0% and macroalbuminuria was present in 0.7% of the population.

- 64% of people with microalbuminuria and 76% of those with macroalbuminuria had co-existent hypertension (Atkins, et al., 2004).

- Abnormal glucose tolerance (diabetes, impaired fasting glucose, or impaired glucose tolerance) was found in 52% of people with micro-albuminuria and 43% of those with macroalbuminuria.

Prevalence of CKD in Asian countries

Estimation of GFR in Asian populations

- Equations to derive eGFR from serum creatinine, such as the MDRD equation, were originally developed in a non-Asian CKD population. Therefore, the validity of using these equations to esti-mate GFR needs to be further assessed in Asian populations.

China and Taiwan

- The prevalence of impaired GFR (<60mL/min/1.73m2) increased with increasing age (0.6% at age 18–39 years, 1.6% at age 40–59 years, 4.6% at age 60–69 years, and 11.8% at age 70 years or older) (Zhang & Rothenbacher, 2008).

- After adjustment for age, independent factors associated with impaired GFR were hypertension for ≥10 years, a history of cardio-vascular disease, HDL level <1.0mmol/L, living in a rural area, and consumption of nephrotoxic medications.

- Diabetes and hypertension were independent factors associated with albuminuria and the risk increased with a longer duration of these diseases.

- Consumption of herbs containing aristolochic acid accounted for two fifths of those taking nephrotoxic medications in the Beijing study (Zhang & Rothenbacher, 2008). In Taiwan, regular users of Chinese herbal medicines had a 20% increased risk of developing CKD (Wen, et al., 2008).

- Comparison of the Beijing data with NHANES data showed that Chinese living in Beijing had a lower prevalence of CKD, albuminu-ria, or impaired GFR than American whites, African Americans, and Hispanics (Xu, et al., 2008). This may be partly explained by the lower prevalence of hypertension, diabetes, hyperlipidaemia, and overweight in the Beijing Chinese.

Table 2.3 Estimated prevalence of CKD in Asian countries, derived from population-based surveys

Country	Study	Reference	Study design, number of participants (n), age group comments	Prevalence of CKD Stage (%)							
				1-5	3-5	1-4	1	2	3	4	5
China	Beijing population study	Zhang, et al., 2008	A representative sample of 13,925 adults aged ≥18 years from greater Beijing (including urban and rural households).	14.0	6.5	14.0	7.4	4.7	1.8	0	0
China	InterASIA	Chen, et al., 2005	A nationally representative sample of 15,540 adults aged from 35–74 years in 2000–2001.	NR	2.53 (1.31 male; 3.82 female)	NR	NR	NR	NR	NR	NR
Thailand	InterASIA	Perkovic, et al., 2008	A population representative sample of 5,146 adults aged ≥35 years.	NR	NR	NR	NR	NR	13.2 (MDRD)	0.61 (MDRD)	NR
Taiwan	MJ Health Management Institution prospective cohort study	Wen, et al., 2008	462,293 adults aged ≥20 years participating in a screening programme run by a private firm, from 1994–2006.	11.93	NR	NR	1.02	3.79	6.81	0.22	0.10
Taiwan	National Health Interview Survey	Hsu, et al., 2006	Nationally representative cross-sectional survey of 6,001 non-institutionalized civilians. Study conducted in 2001 and 2002.	NR	6.9	NR	NR	NR	NR	NR	NR
Japan	Nationwide study	Imai, et al., 2007	527,594 adults aged ≥20 years who received annual health checks as part of community-based, company-based, or hospital-based health check programme from 2000–2004 in seven Japanese prefectures (Hokkaido, Fukushima, Ibaraki, Tokyo, Osaka, Fukuoka, Okinawa).	NR	18.7	NR	NR	NR	18.5	0.2	NR
Japan	Okinawa	Iseki, et al., 2007	Mass screening of 154,019 participants in Okinawa in 2003.	NR	15.1	NR	NR	NR	NR	NR	NR

NR=not reported

- Awareness of CKD in those with impaired GFR was low. Overall, only 3.5% of affected participants knew of their disorder in the Taiwanese cohort study (Wen, et al., 2008). Low awareness was also found in the study by Hsu et al. (Hsu, et al., 2006); only 8.0%, 25.0%, and 71.4% of those with CKD stages 3, 4, and 5, respectively, knew of their kidney disease. A total of 7.9% of those with CKD in the Beijing study were aware they had the disorder (Zhang & Rothenbacher, 2008).

- After follow-up for a median of 7.5 years, those with CKD had a 83% higher all-cause mortality and a 100% higher cardiovascular mortality than those with no CKD (Wen, et al., 2008).

Japan

- Comorbidity of hypertension and diabetes increased as the eGFR declined (Imai, et al., 2007).

- It has been postulated that the high prevalence of CKD in the Japanese population compared to other populations was because the Japanese population has >20% aged >60 years and the normal GFR range is lower in Japanese compared to Caucasians because of smaller kidney size (Imai, et al., 2007).

Prevalence of CKD in ethnic minorities in the West

Canada (Gao, et al., 2007)

- The prevalence of impaired GFR ($<60mL/min/1.73m^2$) was higher in those who were non-First Nations.

- However, the prevalence of severe CKD ($<30mL/min/1.73m^2$) was approximately 2-fold higher in the First Nations group.

- In both First Nations and non-First Nations people, the prevalence of CKD increased with age.

- First Nations people with CKD were significantly younger (median age 60 vs 71 years), were more likely to have diabetes, and live in rural and poor households.

Table 2.4 Estimated prevalence of CKD in ethnic minorities in the West, derived from population-based surveys

Country	Study	Reference	Study design, number of participants (n), age group, comments	Prevalence of CKD stage (%). Minority data are in bold, non-minority data are in italics.							
				1-5	3-5	1-4	1	2	3	4	5
Canada	Alberta provincial study	Gao, et al., 2007	Adults ≥20 years with at least one outpatient serum creatinine level done in 2003–2004. Data were obtained from six out of the nine geographic regions in Alberta province. First Nations (indigenous) classification was obtained from the federal registry. n=658,664 non-First Nations and n=15,989 First Nations people. Urine markers of kidney damage were not examined.	NR	**5.95,** *6.75**	NR	NR	NR	**5.07,** *6.31**	**0.59,** *0.38**	**0.29,** *0.06**
US	NHANES 1999–2004	Coresh, et al., 2007; USRDS, 2007	Nationally representative, cross-sectional continuous survey of the civilian non-institutionalized population aged ≥20 years.	NR	**8.8 (African American),** *7.2 (non Hispanic white)**	NR	NR	NR	NR	NR	NR
US	REGARDS (Reasons for Geographic and Racial Differences in Stroke) Cohort Study.	McClellan, et al., 2006	Nationally representative, population-based cohort of individuals who are ≥45 years, n=20,667.	NR	**33.7 (black),** *49.9 (white)*	NR	NR	NR	NR	NR	NR

* p <0.05; NR=not reported

United States

- From NHANES 1999–2004, the prevalence of low GFR (<60mL/min/1.73m^2) was significantly lower and the prevalence of albuminuria was significantly higher in non-Hispanics African Americans and Mexican Americans compared to non-Hispanic whites (Coresh, et al., 2007).

- In those with a low GFR in the REGARDS study (McClellan, et al., 2006), after adjusting for age, gender, hypertension, diabetes, previous stroke or myocardial infarction, region, and smoking status, the odds of a low GFR in blacks compared to whites remained significantly less than 1.0 until GFR declined below 20mL/min/1.73m^2. However, at GFR from 10–19mL/min/1.73m^2, the odds ratio was 1.73 (95% CI 1.02–2.94) and with GFR <10mL/min/1.73m^2, the odds ratio was 4.19 (95% CI 1.90–9.24).

- Financially disadvantaged groups had higher prevalence of GFR <60mL/min/1.73 m^2 (White, et al., 2008). In non-Hispanic whites, the odds ratio for the lowest vs highest quartile of income was 1.86 (95% CI 1.27–2.72). Unemployment was a more important factor in non-Hispanic blacks and Mexican Americans; the odds ratios of CKD for unemployed vs employed were 2.89 for blacks (95% CI 1.53–5.46) and 6.62 for Mexican Americans (95% CI 1.94–22.64). Multivariate analysis of the association between poverty and albuminuria showed that in the poor, the odds ratio for microalbuminuria in blacks compared to whites was 1.33 (95% CI 1.11–1.60) and the odds ratio for macroalbuminuria was 1.98 (95% CI 1.28–3.06).

Australia

- There has not been a national survey on the prevalence of CKD in indigenous people. The data come from cross-sectional surveys done in different Aboriginal communities. In a remote Aboriginal island community in northern Australia, 487 adults aged ≥18 years were screened (89% of the population) (Hoy, et al., 1998). A total of 26% of adults had microalbuminuria and 24% had overt albuminuria when screened in 1992–5.

- In this population, the ACR correlated with the presence of scabies, past post-streptococcal glomerulonephritis (PSGN), increasing body weight, blood pressure, glucose, insulin, lipid levels, and heavy alcohol drinking.

- A survey done in a remote coastal community of 237 adults aged ≥18 years (53% of the population) showed a crude prevalence of microalbuminuria of 31% and a prevalence of overt albuminuria of 13%; the prevalence of GFR <60mL/min/1.73m^2 was 12% (McDonald, et al., 2003).

- From an analysis of the 2006 census results, indigenous people were (Pink & Allbon, 2008):

  - Three times more likely than non-indigenous people to report themselves as having diabetes.

  - One and a half times more likely to report hypertension.

  - Twice more likely to report regular cigarette smoking.

  - In women, 1.5 times more likely to be overweight or obese than other Australians.

- These comorbidities, coupled with possible biologic factors such as reduced glomerular number at birth and other factors such as socio-economic disadvantage, poor access to health care, and poor cross-cultural communication, may cause the disparity in CKD prevalence in indigenous people compared to other Australians.

Prevalence of CKD in developing countries
Pakistan and India

- Note that the use of 24h urine collection for determining creatinine clearance has the potential for overestimation of GFR because of urine sample under-collection.

- Details of study methods were very brief in some reports (Mani, 2003, 2005). Note that this particular study was not designed primarily to be a prevalence study so not all participants had eGFR.

- In the Delhi study, the mean age of patients affected with CKD was 59 years, and 63% of the CKD was due to diabetes and hypertension (Agarwal, et al., 2005).

Table 2.5 Estimated prevalence of CKD in developing countries, derived from population-based surveys

Country	Study	Reference	Study design, number of participants (n), age group, comments	Prevalence of CKD stage (%)							
				1–5	3–5	1–4	1	2	3	4	5
Pakistan	Community-based sampling	Jafar, et al., 2005	Cross-sectional study of 295 adults aged ≥40 years, which was a representative random sample of households in the metropolitan city of Karachi. GFR was determined by creatinine clearance derived from 24-hour urine collections.	NR	29.9 (26.7 males, 32.5 females)	NR	NR	NR	NR	NR	NR
India	Chronic renal failure prevention programme	Mani, 2003, 2005	Prevention programme run by Kidney Help Trust of Chennai. The initial study was by questionnaire survey and urinalysis of all people ≥5 years, in a population of 25,000 living in rural villages and hamLets located 50km from Chennai. There was 89.6% participation in the original survey. The survey was then extended to adjacent villages (new population of 21,496).	*Original population: 0.86; *New population: 1.39	NR	NR	NR	NR	NR	NR	NR
India	Delhi study	Agarwal, et al., 2005	Multistage cluster sampling within the Southern zones of Delhi. n=4,712. CKD was defined as a serum creatinine >1.8mg/dL, with chronicity defined as persistence of creatinine >1.8mg/dL after three months in the absence of reversible causes.	†0.78	NR	NR	NR	NR	NR	NR	NR
India	Prospective study in hospitals	Dash & Agarwal, 2006	Prospective study in 48 hospitals distributed throughout India, analyzing all prospective investigations done over a 1–3 month period. n=4,172 CKD patients identified.	†0.8	NR	NR	NR	NR	NR	NR	NR

Table 2.5 (Continued) Estimated prevalence of CkD in developing countries, derived from population-based surveys

Country	Study	Reference	Study design, number of participants (n), age group, comments	Prevalence of CKD stage (%)							
				1–5	3–5	1–4	1	2	3	4	5
Vietnam	Population-based survey in six villages	Ito, et al., 2008	Six villages in the Hoai Duc District, Hatay Province, located ~20km west of Hanoi, were studied over a period of 40 days in 2006. n=8,505 adults >40 years. eGFR was estimated using the CG equation.	NR	3.1	NR	NR	NR	NR	NR	NR
Mexico	City of Morelia study	Amato, et al., 2005	Population-based, cross-sectional survey conducted in city of Morelia in a random sample of adults aged ≥18 years. n=3,564. Morelia was a typical Mexican city. Study was conducted in 1999–2000. eGFR was estimated using the CG equation.	NR	8.5	NR	NR	NR	8.1	0.3	0.1
Mexico	The Mexican Health Survey 2000	Rosas, et al., 2005	National, cross-sectional health survey performed in 2000. n=46,523 adults aged 20–69 years. Urine was analyzed once only with a random spot urine and proteinuria was present if dipstick-positive.	Proteinuria 9.2	NR	NR	NR	NR	NR	NR	NR
Chile	First National Health Survey Chile 2003 (NHS 2003)	Escobar, et al., 2006	Nationally representative sample of 3,619 adults ≥17 years. Urine was analyzed once only with a random spot urine and proteinuria was present if dipstick-positive.	Proteinuria 14.0	NR	NR	NR	NR	5.7	0.2	NR
Democratic Republic of Congo	Pilot study in Kinshasa	Sumaili, et al., 2009	Cross-sectional study, 10 out of 35 health zones were sampled randomly, with further multistage sampling of adults ≥20 years. n=500 (91% participation).	12.4	8.0	NR	2.0	2.4	7.8	0	0.2

* CKD defined as GFR <80mL/min/1.73 m²; †CKD defined as serum creatinine >1.8mg/dL for at least three months; NR=not reported

Vietnam (Ito, et al., 2008)

◆ Similar to the findings in other countries, the independent risk factors for CKD were age and hypertension.

◆ There was a low prevalence of diabetes in this predominantly rural population.

◆ Malnutrition rather than obesity was an independent risk factor for CKD.

Mexico (Amato, et al., 2005)

◆ Only 11.1% of people with GFR <60mL/min/1.73m^2 were aware of their kidney disorder.

◆ Factors that were significantly associated with impaired GFR were:

  • Alcohol and cigarette consumption.

  • Female gender.

  • Age >65 years.

  • Educational level lower than primary school.

  • Low income.

Prevalence of proteinuria in Latin American countries, derived from population-based surveys

◆ Results based on a single random spot urine analysis with a dipstick need confirmation because:

  • Urinary protein excretion is variable from day to day.

  • The dipstick measurement is only semi-quantitative.

  • The dipstick does not detect microalbuminuria.

Africa

◆ Population-based studies of CKD prevalence are scarce in this region. The Kinshasa pilot study is one of the first to be attempted (Sumaili, et al., 2009) and the results need confirmation.

◆ In this study, hypertension and age were independently associated with CKD stage 3.

◆ Compared to NHANES data, CKD occurred in a younger age group in the Kinshasa study, with more people in the 40–69 year age group.

◆ Proteinuria was present in 18% (by dipstick) and 5% (defined by protein excretion ≥300mg/dL), and was associated with hypertension.

Incidence of CKD in Western countries

◆ In white adults aged 30–74 years living in the US, incidence rates (per 100,000 person-year) were 84, 7, and 11 for all-cause CKD, diabetic or hypertensive CKD, and treated ESRD, respectively (Tarver–Carr, et al., 2002).

◆ In the European PREVEND cohort study (Verhave, et al., 2004), after four years of follow-up:

  • 11.6% had newly diagnosed elevated urinary albumin excretion.

  • 4.2% had new onset of GFR <60mL/min/1.73m^2.

  • Those with new onset low GFR were older and had higher blood pressure, cholesterol, and glucose levels at baseline, but were no different in body mass index (BMI) to those who did not have reduced GFR at follow-up.

  • Baseline albuminuria was an independent predictor of the development of reduced GFR.

◆ In the Australian AusDiab kidney study (Atkins, et al., 2004; Barr, et al., 2005):

  • The annual incidence of impaired GFR (<60mL/min/1.73m^2) was 0.9% per year.

  • Females had an incidence of 1.3% and males 0.4% per year overall.

  • In females, the incidence in the 50–59 year age group (1.7%) was 3-fold higher compared to those <50 years, and there was another 3-fold rise in incidence in females aged ≥70 years (to 6.3%). In males, the incidence rose in those aged ≥70 years (4.6%).

  • The incidence of impaired GFR was elevated by 2-fold in people with diabetes or with impaired glucose tolerance compared to those without any problem with glucose tolerance or with impaired fasting glucose.

  • Incidence of impaired GFR was about 3-fold greater in those with hypertension compared to those with normal blood pressure.

- The overall annual incidence of albuminuria was 0.8% (1.0% in males and 0.6% in females).
- The incidence of albuminuria was 5-fold higher in those with diabetes and 3-fold higher in those with hypertension.

Incidence of CKD in ethnic minorities in the West

- In the US, a prospective study of 9,082 participants in NHANES II followed for 12–16 years showed that the incidence of all-cause CKD was 2.7-fold increased in African American adults compared to whites (Tarver–Carr, et al., 2002).
- Adjustment for sociodemographic factors, including poverty, education, and marital status, explained 12% of the excess risk.
- Lifestyle factors such as smoking, BMI, alcohol, and physical activity accounted for 32% of excess risk.
- Clinical factors, including diabetes, hypertension, cardiovascular disease, and cholesterol level, accounted for 44% of the excess risk.
- When all the above risk factors were used for adjustment, the relative risk for CKD in African Americans was still 1.95 (95% CI 1.05–3.63), suggesting that ethnicity also was a risk factor.
- Indigenous Australians, the Aboriginal and Torres Strait Islander people comprise 2.5% of the total Australian population; 75% live in capital cities or major regional areas, and 25% live in remote areas (Pink & Allbon, 2008).
- There is little national information about the incidence of pre-dialysis CKD in these people. There is a high prevalence of streptococcal skin infections and PSGN in Aboriginal children living in remote communities. A study following children in one such community for 14.6 years after the occurrence of an epidemic of PSGN showed that after childhood PSGN, the odds ratios for overt albuminuria and any degree of albuminuria on follow-up were 6.1 (95% CI 2.2–16.9) and 3.2 (95% CI 1.7–6.2), respectively (White, et al., 2001).

Prevalence of treated ESRD

Table 2.6 Prevalence of treated ESRD

Country	Registry, reference	Prevalence (pmp), (year)
US	USRDS (2007)	1569, (2005)
UK	European Renal Association–European Dialysis and Transplant Association (ERA-EDTA) (2006)	704.0, (2006)
Italy	European Renal Association–European Dialysis and Transplant Association (ERA-EDTA) (2006)	878.9, (2006)
Norway	European Renal Association–European Dialysis and Transplant Association (ERA-EDTA) (2006)	762.5, (2006)
Australia and New Zealand	Australia and New Zealand Dialysis and Transplant Registry (ANZDATA) (McDonald, et al., 2008a)	778, (2006)

US (2007)

+ In 2005, the median age for people with ESRD was 58.6 years.

+ The prevalence was 1,905 and 1,291 per million population (pmp) in males and females, respectively.

+ Those aged ≥65 years contributed nearly 36% of the prevalent ESRD population.

+ By primary diagnosis, adjusted prevalence (pmp) was 578 for diabetes, 382.7 for hypertension, 254.4 for glomerulonephritis, and 73.3 for cystic kidney disease.

+ The prevalence for diabetes has plateaued since 2000; between 1995 and 2000, the prevalence had increased by 39%, and between 2000 and 2005, it increased by 15.6%.

Minorities in the US

+ In 2005, the prevalence pmp was:
  • 1,151 in whites.
  • 4.2-fold higher for African Americans.
  • 2.3-fold higher for Native Americans.

- Between 2000 and 2005, the prevalence increased by 15% for whites, 8–9% for African Americans and Asians, but fell by 1.1% for Native Americans. The prevalent rate in 2005 for Hispanic people was 47% higher than for non-Hispanic patients. In the last 10 years, the prevalence in Hispanics rose by about 40% compared to an increase of 34% for non-Hispanic people.

- Despite the higher incidence of ESRD in minorities, there appears to be a survival advantage in minorities once they have progressed to ESRD. For example, the USRDS showed that in African Americans and non-white people, respectively, the odds ratios of cardiovascular death within one year of starting dialysis were 0.84 (95% CI 0.80–0.88) and 0.66 (95% CI 0.60–0.73) compared to whites.

- In the Dialysis Outcomes and Practice Patterns study (DOPPS), there was a trend towards better survival in Hispanic patients (hazard ratio for mortality 0.86; 95% CI 0.72–1.03) (Robinson, et al., 2006).

- This apparent survival advantage once people have started on dialysis continues to be a paradox. It may be related to younger age or slightly higher BMI on arrival at ESRD in African Americans (Agodoa, et al., 2007).

- It may also occur because in some minorities, there is a higher risk of mortality in the earlier stages of CKD. Analysis of NHANES III showed that blacks with CKD aged ≤65 years had a 78% higher risk of death (hazard ratio 1.78; 95% CI 1.14–2.78) compared to whites of the same age with CKD (Mehrotra, et al., 2008). The hazard ratio for Mexican Americans in the study was not statistically significant from that of whites.

Australia and New Zealand (McDonald, et al., 2008b)

- Prevalence has more than tripled from 246 pmp in 1983 to 778 pmp in 2006. Factors contributing to this rise are:
  - An ageing population.
  - An increasing acceptance of older people into RRT programmes.
  - The increasing prevalence of diabetes mellitus.
  - Improved survival rates.

- Analysis of trends in causes of treated ESRD from 1981 to 2003 shows (Australian Institute of Health and Welfare, 2005):
  - Glomerulonephritis accounted for 39% of prevalent cases and numbers are still increasing slowly.
  - Diabetic nephropathy accounted for 16% of prevalent cases of treated ESRD.
  - The prevalence of nephropathy due to type 1 diabetes increased 5-fold since 1981 to 33 and 23 pmp in males and females, respectively, while the prevalence due to type 2 diabetes increased greatly by 95-fold and 59-fold, respectively, to 95 pmp in males and 59 pmp in females.
  - Hypertensive nephropathy accounted for 8% of prevalent cases of treated ESRD; the prevalence increased almost 4-fold from 1981 to 2003.

Incidence of treated ESRD

US

- The annual incidence (adjusted for age, sex, and race) of treated ESRD (as reported by USRDS) is defined as the number of people in the population reported as accepted for RRT in a year, compared to the general population size at the start of the year (expressed as pmp).
- In 2005, the incidence was 347 pmp; the median age of people starting treatment was 64.6 years (USRDS, 2007).
- The ESRD incidence has remained relatively stable since 2000.
- Incident rates were 434 and 281 pmp for males and females, respectively.
- Incident rates were:
  - 152 pmp for diabetes as the primary diagnosis (a rate that has stayed stable since 2001).
  - 94 pmp for hypertension (a rate that has slightly decreased since 2003).
  - 26.5 pmp for glomerulonephritis (this rate decreased 6% from 2004).

Minorities in the US

◆ Despite the lower prevalence of CKD in minorities in the US, paradoxically, the incidence of treated ESRD is dramatically higher in these minorities. In 2005, the incident rates pmp were:

  • 268 for whites.

  • 3.7-fold higher for African Americans.

  • 1.9-fold higher for Native Americans.

  • 1.3-fold higher for Asian Americans than for whites (USRDS, 2007).

◆ The incident rate for Hispanic patients was 1.5 times the incident rate for non-Hispanic patients.

◆ From 1995 to 2005, the age-adjusted ESRD incidence increased, but the rate of increase slowed from 1998 to 2005 for both blacks and whites (Burrows, et al., 2008).

◆ For Native Americans, Hispanics, and Asians, the incidence decreased from 1999–2000 through to 2005.

◆ To find out why ESRD incidence was higher in African Americans despite a lower prevalence of CKD stages 1–4, Newsome et al. (2008) analyzed the records of 127,736 people aged ≥65 years hospitalized with myocardial infarction in 1994–95, and then followed for ten years. The aim was to determine if African Americans had higher rates of progression to ESRD or whether whites died before developing ESRD. African Americans had a significantly increased risk of incident ESRD over ten years compared to whites (hazard ratio 1.90, 95% CI 1.78–2.03), and this increased risk was present regardless of the baseline eGFR. The hazard ratio for death before ESRD for African Americans compared to whites was 1.03 (95% CI 1.00–1.05).

◆ A similar analysis was performed in Hispanics and non-Hispanics aged ≥20 years who had CKD stages 3–4 (Peralta, et al., 2006). After adjustment for potential confounders, Hispanics had an increased risk of progression to ESRD (hazard ratio 1.33, 95% CI 1.17–1.52), but a lower risk of cardiovascular events and death. Therefore, there is higher rate of progression to ESRD in African Americans and Hispanics compared to whites.

◆ The effects of poverty and race on ESRD incidence were examined by Volkova et al. (2008). Neighbourhood poverty was associated with increased ESRD incidence and the poorest neighbourhoods had more than three times the incident rate of the well-off areas. As the degree of poverty increased, there was a greater increase in ESRD incident rates in blacks compared to whites.

Europe

The age- and gender-adjusted incident rates are shown in Table 2.7 for representative countries from Western Europe, from data from ERA-EDTA (2006).

Table 2.7 Adjusted ESRD incidence pmp at day 91

Country	Total	Diabetes as primary diagnosis	Hypertension as primary diagnosis	Glomerulonephritis as primary diagnosis
UK	100.4	21.7	5.0	11.6
Italy	104.6	16.8	15.9	10.4
Norway	96.1	16.2	25.8	19.6

◆ Incidence for all-cause ESRD and diabetic ESRD in Northern Europe have stabilized since 2000, but have increased in Southern Europe since 2002 (by 8.8% and 12.4%, respectively) (Jager & Van Dijk, 2007).

◆ The lower incidence of treated ESRD and the lower proportion of incident RRT patients with diabetes or hypertension in Western Europe vs the US have been noted previously.

◆ Hallan et al. (2006b) from Norway reported on eight years of follow-up of 3,069 people with CKD (HUNT II study). Only 38 people (1.2%) progressed to ESRD.
  - In those with baseline GFR 30–60mL/min/1.73m^2, the ESRD incident rate and cardiovascular mortality rate per 100 person-years were 0.1 and 4.2, respectively.
  - In those with baseline GFR <30mL/min/1.73m^2, the incident rates were 2.6 and 10.1, respectively.

◆ When compared to Norwegian patients (Hallan, et al., 2006a), US white patients had a 2.5-fold increased risk of progression to treated ESRD from CKD stages 3–4; this risk was 2.0-fold for those without diabetes, 2.8-fold for those with diabetes, 1.7-fold for those <60 years old, 3.0-fold for those ≥60 years old, 3.5-fold for females, and 1.9-fold for males (Hallan, et al., 2006a). Earlier nephrologist referral and lower prevalence of obesity in Norway may explain the differences between the renal data from the two countries.

Australia and New Zealand

- ◆ ANZDATA showed that in 2006, the age-standardized incidence of people treated for ESRD was 115 pmp and the median age of people starting treatment was 63.2 years (McDonald, et al., 2008a).

- ◆ Overall, there has been a steady increase in incidence starting from the 1980s. Back in 1981, the annual incidence was 40 pmp.

- ◆ In 2006, the largest increases in incidence were in those aged ≥65 years of age.

- ◆ A total of 32% of incident cases were caused by diabetic nephropathy, 23% by glomerulonephritis, and 15% by hypertension.

- ◆ The incidence of treated ESRD caused by type 1 diabetes has increased only slightly since 1981, but the incidence caused by type 2 diabetes has increased steeply.

Minorities in Australia

- ◆ In 2005, 207 out of 2,378 people newly registered with ANZDATA (8.7%) were Aboriginal or Torres Strait Islander (McDonald, et al., 2008c).

  - • The age-standardized incident rate pmp for indigenous people starting treatment for ESRD was 741.

  - • The incidence ratio for indigenous compared to other ethnic groups was 6.8.

  - • The median age of new indigenous patients was younger (55 years).

  - • The incidence ratio of indigenous compared to non-indigenous people was 17.6 for the 45–54 year age group and 14.0 for the 55–64 year age group (Australian Institute of Health and Welfare, 2005).

- Since 1991, there was an annual average increase in the incidence of treated ESRD of 13% per year for indigenous people compared to 5% per year in non-indigenous people (Australian Institute of Health and Welfare, 2005).

- Compared to non-indigenous people, the ESRD incidence was higher in indigenous Australians living in remote areas (26 times higher) and in very remote areas (12 times higher) (Pink & Allbon, 2008).

  - In major cities and large regional areas, indigenous people still had 4–5 times the incidence of ESRD of non-indigenous people.

  - Compared to non-indigenous new patients, there was an increased proportion of indigenous people reporting diabetes as the primary cause of the renal disease (>58% vs 22% in non-indigenous people).

Treated ESRD in developing countries

Africa

In the Democratic Republic of Congo, the primary renal diseases leading to ESRD were (Krzesinski, et al., 2007):

- Glomerulonephritis (35%).
- Hypertension (30%).
- Diabetes (25%).

In North Africa, the incidence of ESRD pmp ranged from 34 in Algeria to 200 in Libya (Barsoum, 2003). The primary renal diseases were:

- Interstitial nephritis (14–32%).
- Glomerulonephritis (11–24%).
- Diabetes (5–20%).
- Hypertensive nephrosclerosis (5–21%).

In Egypt:

- The prevalence of diabetic nephropathy in ESRD patients enrolled in the Egyptian renal data system increased from 8.9% in 1996 to 14.5% in 2001 (Afifi, et al., 2004).

- Hypertension and obstructive uropathy were also important causes of ESRD.

- In North Africa, there is a high prevalence of schistosomiasis leading to obstruction. Obstructive uropathy accounted for 7% of people on dialysis in Egypt.

In Tunisia:

- The incidence of ESRD rose by an average of 9.6% per year over ten years, from 81.6 pmp in 1992–3 to 158.8 pmp in 2000–2001 (Counil, et al., 2008).

- The annual average increase in incidence for diabetic nephropathy was 16.1% per year, 7.6% per year for hypertensive and other reno-vascular disease, and 10.4% for tubulointerstitial disease.

The prevalence of dialysis-treated ESRD in North Africa ranged from 30.0 pmp in Libya to 430.0 pmp in Tunisia (Barsoum, 2006), with haemodialysis as the main modality and dialysis pool size reflecting relative national wealth.

In India:

- A large population-based survey of 572,029 people in Bhopal established that the incidence of ESRD was 232 pmp, with an average age 47 years and 58% were males (Modi & Jha, 2006).

- A total of 44% of ESRD was caused by diabetic nephropathy.

- Previously, chronic glomerulonephritis and interstitial nephritis were the main causes of ESRD.

- It is estimated that less than 10% of people with ESRD in India receive RRT; of those who start dialysis, 70% die or stop treatment within three months because of the cost, and only 5% receive a transplant (Sakhuja & Sud, 2003).

Global cost of CKD and ESRD

The preceding sections have revealed the extent of the global problem of increasing prevalence of CKD and ESRD. Already, it is apparent that there are socio-economic and ethnic disparities in kidney disease, both in the occurrence of disease as well as access to care, and the burden of disease is falling on those least able to cope (Agodoa, et al., 2005).

In 2005, the total Medicare programme expenditure in the US was $331.4 billion. CKD (including ESRD) expenditure accounted for 27.6% of total Medicare expenditure and 35.5% of expenditure for the medically disabled or indigent who had dual Medicare and Medicaid coverage (USRDS, 2007). ESRD alone accounted for 6.4% of the Medicare programme or $21.3 billion in 2005. This expenditure more than tripled since 1991. ESRD Medicare costs are forecast to rise at 7.7% annually to reach $28.3 billion by 2010 (Xue, et al., 2001). Medicare covers people aged 65 years or older or with a qualifying disability. People not covered by Medicare are not entitled to Medicare coverage until three months after the onset of ESRD. This makes it harder for people who are either uninsured with private health insurance or underinsured to have the diagnosis and treatment of CKD at the pre-dialysis stage.

In Australia, in 2000–2001, CKD total expenditure was $647 million or 1.3% of total recurrent health expenditure (Australian Institute of Health and Welfare, 2005). ESRD care is predominantly through publicly funded facilities and there is universal health insurance through the Australian Medicare system. Projected annual heath care costs for treating all cases of ESRD are expected to rise from $559.5 million in 2004 to $4.26–4.52 billion in 2010 (Cass, et al., 2006).

In the UK, in 2002, it was estimated that 1.5% of total health spending was used for RRT, a cost of £32,500 per patient per year (US$ 53,279) (Nicholson & Roderick, 2007). The percent of the total health care budget spent on ESRD was 1.8% in Italy (Pontoriero, 2007), 1.3% in France (Durand–Zaleski, et al., 2007), and 1.8% in Belgium (Van Biesen, et al., 2007). The estimated treatment cost of renal failure caused by diabetic nephropathy in Germany in 2002 was €7,862–10,223 per patient per year (Happich, et al., 2008). Apart from direct costs, CKD has other flow-on costs. A German study on the effect of different stages of CKD on the in-hospital costs of patients with coronary heart disease found that costs increased by €18 with each 1mL/min reduction in eGFR (Meyer, et al., 2008).

It was estimated that in 2005, the number of patients with ESRD was 1.9 million worldwide and this number was increasing by 6–7% per year compared to the 1.2% annual growth rate for the total global population (Grassmann, et al., 2006). A total of 40% of dialysis patients lived in low- or middle-income countries. In 2001, a cost estimate of global maintenance ESRD therapy, excluding renal transplantation, was US$ 70–75 billion (Lysaght, 2002). The total global cumulative cost for dialysis from 2001–10 was estimated to be US$ 1,088 billion. By 2030, more than 70% of people with ESRD will reside in developing countries, which account for only 15% of the total global economy (Barsoum, 2005). These countries spend 0.8–4.0% of gross domestic product on health care, compared to 10–15% in developed countries (Jafar, 2006). These areas are the regions in which the most growth in prevalence of diabetes is anticipated. In 2007, 246 million people worldwide aged 20–79 years (5.9%) had diabetes, and this will increase to 7.1% (380 million) by 2025 (International Diabetes Federation, 2006). Regionally, there will be an increase of 80% in Africa, 81% in the Eastern Mediterranean and Middle East, 101% in South and Central America, 73% in South East Asia, and 48% in the Western Pacific Region, compared to a 21% rise in Europe and 43% increase in North America. Therefore, innovative international schemes are urgently needed to prevent, detect, and treat CKD (Atkins, 2005; Schieppati & Remuzzi, 2004).

References

Afifi, A., El Setouhy, M., El Sharkawy, M., Ali, M., Ahmed, H., El-Menshawy, O., Masoud, W., 2004. Diabetic nephropathy as a cause of end-stage renal disease in Egypt: a six-year study. *Eastern Mediterrean Health Journal*, 10(4–5), pp.620–6.

Agarwal, S., Dash, S., Irshad, M., Raju, S., Singh, R., Pandey, R., 2005. Prevalence of chronic renal failure in adults in Delhi, India. *Nephrology Dialysis Transplantation*, 20(8), pp.1638–42.

Agodoa, L., Norris, K., Pugsley, D., 2005. The disproportionate burden of kidney disease in those who can least afford it. *Kidney International*, 68(Suppl 97), S1–3.

Agodoa, L., Eggers, P., 2007. Racial and ethnic disparities in end-stage kidney failure-survival paradoxes in African Americans. *Seminars in Dialysis*, 20(6), pp.577–85.

Amato, D., Alvarez-Aguilar, C., Castañeda-Limones, R., Rodriguez, E., Avila–Diaz, M., Arreola, F., Gomez, A., Ballesteros, H., Becerril, R., Paniagua, R., 2005. Prevalence of chronic kidney disease in an urban Mexican population. *Kidney International Suppl*, (97), S11–7.

Atkins, R., Polkinghorne, K., Briganti, E., Shaw, J., Zimmet, P., Chadban, S., 2004. Prevalence of albuminuria in Australia: the AusDiab Kidney Study. *Kidney International Suppl*, 92, S22–4.

Atkins, R., 2005. The changing patterns of chronic kidney disease: The need to develop strategies for prevention relevant to different regions and countries. *Kidney International*, 68(Suppl 98), S83–5.

Australian Institute of Health and Welfare, 2005. *Chronic kidney disease in Australia 2005*. Canberra: Australian Institute of Health and Welfare.

Barr, E., Magliano, D., Zimmet, P., Polkinghorne, K., Atkins, R., Dunstan, D., Murray, S., Shaw, J. 2006 (Version 2). Background, Chapter One. In: Barr, E., Magliano, D., Zimmet, P., Polkinghorne, K., Atkins, R., Dunstan, D., Murray, S., Shaw, J. *AusDiab 2005. The Australian Diabetes, Obesity and Lifestyle Study. Tracking the Accelerating Epidemic: Its Causes and Outcomes*. Melbourne: The International Diabetes Institute, pp. 1–5.

Barr, E., Magliano, D., Zimmet, P., Polkinghorne, K., Atkins, R., Dunstan, D., Murray, S., Shaw, J. 2006 (Version 2). Chronic kidney diesease, Chapter 6. In: Barr, E., Magliano, D., Zimmet, P., Polkinghorne, K., Atkins, R., Dunstan, D., Murray, S., Shaw, J. *AusDiab 2005. The Australian Diabetes, Obesity and Lifestyle Study. Tracking the Accelerating Epidemic: Its Causes and Outcomes*. Melbourne: International Diabetes Institute, pp. 35–8.

Barsoum, R., 2003. End-stage renal disease in North Africa. *Kidney International*, 63(Suppl 83), S111–4.

Barsoum, R., 2005. Epidemiology of ESRD: a world-wide perpective. In: El-Nahas, M., Barsoum, R,. Dirks, J., Remuzzi, G., eds. *Kidney diseases in the developing world and ethnic minorities*. London: Taylor and Francis, pp.1 13.

Barsoum, R., 2006. Chronic kidney disease in the developing world. *New England Journal of Medicine*, 354(10), pp.997–9.

Burrows, N., Li, Y., Williams, D., 2008. Racial and ethnic differences in trends of end-stage renal disease: United States, 1995–2005. *Advances in Chronic Kidney Disease*, 15(2), pp.147–52.

Cass, A., Chadban, S., Craig, J., Howard, K., McDonald, S., Salkeld, G., White, S. 2006. Economic impact of end-stage kidney disease in Australia. Melbourne: Kidney Health Australia [available at: http://www.kidney.org.au/].

Chen, J., Wildman, R., Gu, D., Kusek, J.W., Spruill, M., Reynolds, K., Liu, D., Hamm, L.L., Whelton, P.K., He, J., 2005. Prevalence of decreased kidney function in Chinese adults aged 35 to 74 years. *Kidney International*, 68(6), pp.2837–45.

Cirillo, M., Laurenzi, M., Mancini, M., Zanchetti, A., Lombardi, C., De Santo, N., 2006. Low glomerular filtration in the population: prevalence, associated disorders, and awareness. *Kidney International*, 70(4), pp.800–6.

Coresh, J., Selvin, E., Stevens, L.A., Manzi, J., Kusek, J.W., Eggers, P., Van Lente, F., Levey, A.S., 2007. Prevalence of Chronic Kidney Disease in the United States. *Journal of the American Medical Association*, 298(17), pp.2038–47.

Counil, E., Cherni, N., Kharrat, M., Achour, A., Trimech, H., 2008. Trends of incident dialysis patients in Tunisia between 1992 and 2001. *American Journal of Kidney Diseases*, 51(2), pp.463–70.

Dash, S., Agarwal, S., 2006. Incidence of chronic kidney disease in India. *Nephrology Dialysis Transplantation*, 21(1), pp.232–3.

de Zeeuw, D., Hillege, H., de Jong, P., 2005. The kidney, a cardiovascular risk marker, and a new target for therapy. *Kidney International Suppl*, 98, S25–9.

Durand–Zaleski, I., Combe, C., Lang, P., 2007. International study of health care organization and financing for end-stage renal disease in France. *International Journal of Health Care Finance and Economics*, 7(2–3), pp.171–83.

Escobar, C., Arce, I., Jara, A., Mezzano, S., Ardiles, L., 2006. Renal health in Chile. *Renal Failure*, 28(8), pp.639–41.

European Renal Association-European Dialysis and Transplant Association Registry, 2006. *ERA-EDTA Registry 2006 Annual Report*. Amsterdam: Academic Medical Centre, Department of Medical Informatics.

Fox, C., Muntner, P., 2008. Trends in diabetes, high cholesterol, and hypertension in chronic kidney disease among U.S. adults: 1988–1994 to 1999–2004. *Diabetes Care*, 31(7), pp.1337–42.

Gansevoort, R., Verhave, J., Hillege, H., Burgerhof, J.G., Bakker, S.J., de Zeeuw, D., de Jong, P.E.; for the PREVEND Study Group, 2005. The validity of screening based on spot morning urine samples to detect subjects with microalbuminuria in the general population. *Kidney International Suppl*, 94, S28–35.

Gao S, Manns B, Culleton B, Tonelli, M., Quan, H., Crowshoe, L., Ghali, W.A., Svenson, L.W., Hemmelgarn, B.R.; Alberta Kidney Disease Network, 2007. Prevalence of chronic kidney disease and survival among aboriginal people. *Journal of the American Society of Nephrology*, 18(11), pp.2953–9.

Glassock, R., Winearls, C., 2008. The global burden of chronic kidney disease: How valid are the estimates? *Nephron Clinical Practice*, 110(1), c39–47.

Grassmann, A., Gioberge, S., Moeller, S., Brown, G., 2006. End-stage renal disease: global demographics in 2005 and observed trends. *Artificial Organs*, 30(12), pp.895–7.

Hallan, S., Coresh, J., Astor, B., Asberg, A., Powe, N.R., Romundstad, S., Hallan, H.A., Lydersen, S., Holmen, J., 2006a. International comparison of the relationship of chronic kidney disease prevalence and ESRD risk. *Journal of the American Society of Nephrology*, 17(8), pp.2275–84.

Hallan, S.I., Dahl, K., Oien, C.M., Grootendorst, D.C., Aasberg, A, Holmen, J., Dekker, F.W., 2006b. Screening strategies for chronic kidney disease in the general population: follow-up of cross sectional health survey. *British Medical Journal*, 333(7577), p.1047.

Happich, M., Landgraf, R., Piehlmeier, W., Falkenstein, P., Stamenitis, S., 2008. The economic burden of nephropathy in diabetic patients in Germany in 2002. *Diabetes Research and Clinical Practice*, 80(1), pp.34–9.

Hoy, W., Mathews, J., McCredie, D., Pugsley, D.J., Hayhurst, B.G., Rees, M., Kile, E., Walker, K.A., Wang, Z., 1998. The multidimensional nature of renal disease: rates and associations of albuminuria in an Australian Aboriginal community. *Kidney International*, 54(4), pp.1296–304.

Hsu, C., Hwang, S., Wen, C., Chang, H.Y., Chen, T., Shiu, R.S., Horng, S.S., Chang, Y.K., Yang, W.C., 2006. High prevalence and low awareness of CKD in Taiwan: a study on the relationship between serum creatinine and awareness from a nationally representative survey. *American Journal of Kidney Diseases*, 48(5), pp.727–38.

Imai, E., Horio, M., Iseki, K., Yamagata, K., Watanabe, T., Hara, S., Ura, N., Kiyohara, Y., Hirakata, H., Moriyama, T., Ando, Y., Nitta, K., Inaguma, D., Narita, I., Iso, H., Wakai, K., Yasuda, Y., Tsukamoto, Y., Ito, S., Makino, H., Hishida, A., Matsuo, S., 2007. Prevalence of chronic kidney disease (CKD) in the Japanese general population predicted by the MDRD equation modified by a Japanese coefficient. *Clinical and Experimental Nephrology*, 11(2), pp.156–63.

International Diabetes Federation, 2006. *Diabetes Atlas*. 3rd ed. Brussels: International Diabetes Federation.

Iseki, K., Kohagura, K., Sakima, A., Iseki, C., Kinjo, K., Ikemiya, Y., Takishita, S., 2007. Changes in the demographics and prevalence of chronic kidney disease in Okinawa, Japan (1993–2003). *Hypertension Research*, 30, pp.55–62.

Ito, J., Dung, D., Vuong, M., Tuyen do, G., Vinh le, D., Huong, N.T., Ngoc, T.B., Ngoc, N.T., Hien, M.T., Hao, D.D., Oanh, L.T., Lieu do, T., Fujisawa, M., Kawabata, M., Shirakawa, T., 2008. Impact and perspective on chronic kidney disease in an Asian developing country: a large-scale survey in north Vietnam. *Nephron Clinical Practice*, 109(1), c25–32.

Jafar, T., Schmid, C., Levey, A., 2005. Serum creatinine as marker of kidney function in South Asians: a study of reduced GFR in adults in Pakistan. *Journal of the American Society of Nephrology*, 16(5), pp.1413–9.

Jafar, T., 2006. The growing burden of chronic kidney disease in Pakistan. *New England Journal of Medicine*, 354(10), pp.995–7.

Jager, K., Van Dijk, P., 2007. Has the rise in the incidence of renal replacement therapy in developed countries come to an end? *Nephrology Dialysis Transplantation*, 22(3), pp.678–80.

Krzesinski, J., Sumaili, E., Cohen, E., 2007. How to tackle the avalanche of chronic kidney disease in sub-Saharan Africa: the situation in the Democratic Republic of Congo as an example. *Nephrology Dialysis Transplantation*, 22(3), pp.332–5.

Levey, A.S., Bosch, J.P., Lewis, J.B., Greene, T., Rogers, N., Roth, D., 1999. A more accurate method to estimate glomerular filtration rate from serum creatinine: a new prediction equation. Modification of Diet in Renal Disease Study Group. *Annals of Internal Medicine*, 130(6), pp.461–70.

Levey, A., Eckardt, K., Tsukumato, Y., Levin, A., Coresh, J., Rossert, J., De Zeeuw, D., Hostetter, T.H., Lameire, N., Eknoyan,, G., 2005. Definition and classification of chronic kidney disease: a global position statement from Kidney Disease: Improving Global Outcome (KDIGO). *Kidney International*, 67(6), pp.2098–100.

Levey, A., Atkins, R., Coresh, J., Cohen, E.P., Collins, A.J., Eckardt, K.U., Nahas, M.E., Jaber, B.L., Jadoul, M., Levin, A., Powe, N.R., Rossert, J., Wheeler, D.C., Lameire, N., Eknoyan, G., 2007a. Chronic kidney disease as a global public health problem: approaches and initiatives–a position statement from Kidney Disease Improving Global Outcomes. *Kidney International*, 72(3), pp.247–59.

Levey, A., Coresh, J., Greene, T., Marsh, J., Stevens, L.A., Kusek, J.W., Van Lente, F.; Chronic Kidney Disease Epidemiology Collaboration, 2007b. Expressing the Modification of Diet in Renal Disease Study equation for estimating glomerular filtration rate with standardized serum creatinine values. *Clinical Chemistry*, 53(4), pp.766–72.

Lysaght, M., 2002. Maintenance dialysis population dynamics: Current trends and long term implications. *Journal of the American Society of Nephrology*, 13(Suppl 1), S37–40.

Mani, M., 2003. Prevention of chronic renal failure at the community level. *Kidney International*, 63(Suppl 83), S86–9.

Mani, M., 2005. Experience with a program for prevention of chronic renal failure in India. *Kidney International*, 67(Suppl 94), S75–8.

McClellan, W., Warnock, D., McClure, L., Campbell, R.C., Newsome, B.B., Howard, V., Cushman, M., Howard, G., 2006. Racial differences in the prevalence of chronic kidney disease among participants in the Reasons for Geographic and Racial Differences in Stroke (REGARDS) Cohort Study. *Journal of the American Society of Nephrology*, 17(6), pp.1710–5.

McDonald, S., Chang, S., Excell, L. 2008a. New patients commencing treatment in 2006. Chapter 2. In: McDonald, S., Chang, S., Excell, L., eds. *ANZDATA Registry Report 2007*. Adelaide: Australia and New Zealand Dialysis and Transplant Registry, pp.2-1 to 2-12.

McDonald, S., Excell, L. 2008b. Stock and flow. Chapter 1. In: McDonald, S., Chang, S., Excell, L., eds. *ANZDATA Registry Report 2007*. Adelaide: Australia and New Zealand Dialysis and Transplant Registry, p.1-1.

McDonald, S., Chang, S. Excell, L. 2008c. New Patients. Appendix II. In: McDonald, S., Chang, S., Excell, L. eds. *ANZDATA Registry Report 2007*. Adelaide: Australia and New Zealand Dialysis and Transplant Registry, pp.1–97.

McDonald, S., Maguire, G., Hoy, W., 2003. Renal function and cardiovascular risk markers in a remote Australian Aboriginal community. *Nephrology Dialysis Transplantation*, 18(8), pp.1555–61.

Mehrotra, R., Kermah, D., Fried, L., Adler, S., Norris, K.. 2008. Racial differences in mortality among those with CKD. *Journal of the American Society of Nephrology*, 19(7), pp.1403–10.

Meyer, A., Bunzemeier, H., Hausberg, M., Walter, M., Roeder, N., Breithardt, G., Reinecke, H., 2008. Impact of different stages of chronic kidney disease on in-hospital costs in patients with coronary heart disease. *Nephrology Dialysis Transplantation*, 23(6), pp.1955–60.

Modi, G., Jha, V., 2006. The incidence of end-stage renal disease in India: a population-based study. *Kidney International*, 70(12), pp.2131–3.

Newsome, B., McClellan, W., Allison, J., Eggers, P.W., Chen, S.C., Collins, A.J., Kiefe, C.I., Coffey, C.S., Warnock, D.G., 2008. Racial differences in the competing risks of mortality and ESRD after acute myocardial infarction. *American Journal of Kidney Diseases*, 52(2), pp.251–61.

Nicholson, T., Roderick, P., 2007. International study of health care organization and financing of renal services in England and Wales. *International Journal of Health Care Finance and Economics*, 7(4), pp.283–99.

Nitsch, D., Felber Dietrich, D., von Eckardstein, A., Gaspoz, J.M., Downs, S.H., Leuenberger, P., Tschopp, J.M., Brandli, O., Keller, R., Gerbase, M.W., Probst–Hensch, N.M., Stutz, E.Z., Ackermann–Liebrich, U.; SAPALDIA team, 2006. Prevalence of renal impairment and its association with cardiovascular risk factors in a general population: results of the Swiss SAPALDIA study. *Nephrology Dialysis Transplantation*, 21(4), pp.935–44.

Otero, A., Gayoso, P., Garcia, F., De Francisco, A.,2005. Epidemiology of chronic renal disease in the Galician popluation: Results of the pilot Spanish EPIRCE study. *Kidney International*, 68(Suppl 99), S16–9.

Peralta, C., Shlipak, M., Fan, D., Ordonez, J., Lash, J.P., Chertow, G.M., Go, A.S., 2006. Risks for end-stage renal disease, cardiovascular events, and death in Hispanic versus non-Hispanic white adults with chronic kidney disease. *Journal of the American Society of Nephrology*, 17(10), pp.2892–9.

Perkovic, V., Cass, A., Patel, A., Suriyawongpaisal, P., Barzi, F., Chadban, S., Macmahon, S., Neal, B.; InterASIA Collaborative Group, 2008. High prevalence of chronic kidney disease in Thailand. *Kidney International*, 73(4), pp.473–9.

Pink, B., Allbon, P., 2008. *The health and welfare of Australia's Aboriginal and Torres Strait Islander peoples 2008*. Report number: ABS catalogue No 4704.0, AIHW catalogue No IHW 21. Canberra: Australian Bureau of Statistics and Australian Institute of Health and Welfare.

Polkinghorne, K., Chadban, S., Atkins, R. 2008. Personal communication.

Pontoriero, G., Pozzoni, P., Del Vecchio, L., Locatelli, F., 2007. International study of health care organization and financing for renal replacement therapy in Italy: an evolving reality. *International Journal of Health Care Finance and Economics*, 7(2–3), pp.201–15.

Robinson, B., Joffe, M., Pisoni, R., Port, F., Feldman, H., 2006. Revisiting survival differences by race and ethnicity among hemodialysis patients: the Dialysis Outcomes and Practice Patterns Study. *Journal of the American Society of Nephrology*, 17(10), pp.2910–8.

Rosas, M., Attie, F., Pastelin, G., Lara, A., Velazquez, O., Tapia–Conyer, R., Martinez–Reding, J., Mendez, A., Lorenzo–Negrete, A., Herrera–Acosta., J., 2000. Prevalance of proteinuria in Mexico: a conjunctive consolidation approach with other cardio-vascular risk factors: the Mexican Health Survey 2000. *Kidney International Suppl*, 97, S112–9.

Sakhuja, V., Sud, K., 2003. End-stage renal disease in India and Pakistan: Burden of disease and management issues. *Kidney International*, 63(Suppl 83), S115–8.

Schena, F., 2000. Epidemiology of end-stage renal disease: International comparisons of renal replacement therapy. *Kidney International*, 57(Suppl 74), S39–45.

Schieppati, A., Remuzzi, G., 2004. Fighting renal diseases in poor countries: Building a global fund with the help of the pharmaceutical industry. *Journal of the American Society of Nephrology*, 15(3), pp.704–7.

Sumaili, E., Krzesinski, J., Zinga, C., Cohen, E.P., Delanaye, P., Munyanga, S.M., Nseka, N.M., 2009. Prevalence of chronic kidney disease in Kinshasa: results of a pilot study from the Democratic Republic of Congo. *Nephrology Dialysis Transplantation*, 24(1), pp.117–22.

Tarver–Carr, M., Powe, N., Eberhardt, M., LaVeist, T.A., Kington, R.S., Coresh, J., Brancati, F.L., 2002. Excess risk of chronic kidney disease among African-American versus white subjects in the United States: a population-based study of potential explanatory factors. *Journal of the American Society of Nephrology*, 13(9), pp.2363–70.

United States Renal Data System, 2007. *Annual data report: Atlas of chronic kidney disease and end-stage renal disease in the United States* 2007. Bethesda: National Institutes of Health, National Institute of Diabetes and Digestive and Kidney Diseases.

United States Renal Data System, 2008. *Annual data report: Atlas of chronic kidney disease and end-stage renal disease in the United States 2008*. Bethesda: National Institutes of Health, National Institute of Diabetes and Digestive and Kidney Diseases.

Van Biesen, W., Lameire, N., Peeters, P., Vanholder, R., 2007. Belgium's mixed private/public health care system and its impact on the cost of end-stage renal disease. *International Journal of Health Care Finance and Economics*, 7(2–3), pp.133–48.

Verhave, J.C., Gansevoort, R.T., Hillege, H.L., Bakker, S.J., De Zeeuw, D., de Jong, P.E., 2004. An elevated urinary albumin excretion predicts de novo development of renal function impairment in the general population. *Kidney International Suppl*, (92), S18–21.

Verhave, J., Hillege, H., Burgerhof, J., Gansevoort, R.T., de Zeeuw, D., de Jong, P.E.; PREVEND Study Group, 2005. The association between atherosclerotic risk factors and renal function in the general population. *Kidney International*, 67(5), pp.1967–73.

Viktorsdottir, O., Palsson, R., Andresdottir, M., Aspelund, T., Gudnason, V., Indridason, O., 2005. Prevalence of chronic kidney disease based on estimated glomerular filtration rate and proteinuria in Icelandic adults. *Nephrology Dialysis Transplantation*, 20(9), pp.1799–807.

Volkova, N., McClellan, W., Klein, M., Flanders, D., Kleinbaum, D., Soucie, J.M., Presley, R., 2008. Neighborhood poverty and racial differences in ESRD incidence. *Journal of the American Society of Nephrology*, 19(25), pp.356–64.

Wen, C., Cheng, T., Tsai, M., Chang, Y.C., Chan, H.T., Tsai, S.P., Chiang, P.H., Hsu, C.C., Sung, P.K., Hsu, Y.H., Wen, S.F., 2008. All-cause mortality attributable to chronic kidney disease: a prospective cohort study based on 462 293 adults in Taiwan. *Lancet*, 371(9631), pp.2173–82.

White, A., Hoy, W., McCredie, D., 2001. Childhood post-streptococcal glomerulone-phritis as a risk factor for chronic renal disease in later life. *Medical Journal of Australia*, 174(10), pp.492–6.

White, S., McGeechan, K., Jones, M., Cass, A., Chadban, S.J., Polkinghorne, K.R., Perkovic, V., Roderick, P.J., 2008. Socioeconomic disadvantage and kidney disease in the United States, Australia, and Thailand. *American Journal of Public Health*, 98(7), pp.1306–13.

Xu, R., Zhang, L., Zhang, P., Wang, F., Zuo, L., Wang, H., 2009. Comparison of the prevalence of chronic kidney disease among different ethnicities: Beijing CKD survey and American NHANES. *Nephrology Dialysis Transplantation*, 24(4), pp.1220–6.

Xue, J., Ma, J., Louis, T., Collins, A., 2001. Forecast of the number of patients with end-stage renal disease in the United States to the year 2010. *Journal of the American Society of Nephrology*, 12(12), pp.2753–8.

Zhang, Q., Rothenbacher, D., 2008. Prevalence of chronic kidney disease in popula-tion-based studies: Systematic review. *BMC Public Health*, 8, pp.117–30.

Zhang, L., Zhang, P., Wang, F., Zuo, L., Zhou, Y, Shi, Y, Li, G., Jiao, S., Liu, Z., Liang, W., Wang, H., 2008. Prevalence and factors associated with CKD: a population study from Beijing. *American Journal of Kidney Diseases*, 51(3), pp.373–84.

Chapter 3

Chronic kidney disease: classification, risk factors, and natural history

Marcellus Assiago, Andrew S. Levey, and Lesley A. Stevens

Introduction

Chronic kidney disease (CKD) is a growing health care concern and public health burden in developed and developing countries. In many countries, CKD prevalence is already high and increasing (see Chapter 1). The natural history of CKD is initially kidney damage, which, if progressive, can lead to a decline in kidney function and ultimately, to kidney failure. CKD is also associated with complications, which include cardiovascular in particular, as well as complications of decreased kidney function, which in their most severe form is known as the uraemic syndrome. There are treatments for each stage of CKD, and therefore, timely detection of CKD and initiation of treatments are important to prevent or slow progression as well as prevent further complications. In this chapter, we review the definition and classification for CKD, its natural history, and risk factors for development, progression, and complications of the disease. Recently, an increased interest has been focused on emerging subsets of the population with a high prevalence of CKD, specifically the elderly. The presence of CKD complicates the management of chronic comorbid diseases, which are also highly prevalent in the elderly. Attention has also been directed towards ethnic and racial minorities as they have unique risk factors for development and progression of CKD.

Definition, classification, and clinical action plan

Definition of CKD

CKD is defined as: kidney damage for at least three months, with or without decreased GFR:

- Pathological abnormalities.
- Markers of kidney damage:
  - Urinary abnormalities (proteinuria).
  - Blood abnormalities (renal tubular syndromes).
  - Imaging abnormalities.
  - Kidney transplantation.
- GFR <60mL/min/1.73m^2 for at least three months, with or without kidney damage.

Kidney damage, even with normal GFR, is defined as CKD for three main reasons:

- Kidney damage may occur before GFR declines.
- Kidney damage portends a worse prognosis for the major outcomes related to CKD.
- Higher levels of kidney damage are associated with a faster decline in GFR, increased risk of kidney failure, and cardiovascular disease (CVD).

Kidney damage

Kidney damage is usually ascertained by measuring markers of damage rather than a kidney biopsy. The most common markers of kidney damage are urine proteins which consist of:

- High molecular weight proteins that are filtered only when the glomerulus is damaged such as albumin.
- Low molecular weight proteins that are filtered normally and incompletely reabsorbed.
- Tubular protein.
- Proteins derived from the lower urinary tract.

Why is albuminuria the principal marker of kidney damage in adults?

- It is a specific sign of glomerular damage.
- In developed countries, diabetes and hypertension are the most common causes of kidney disease. This leads to glomerular damage, which is evident by the presence of albuminuria.

Table 3.1 defines abnormal levels of urine protein and urine albumin according to the method used for collection. Due to the difficulty in collecting a timed urine specimen, it is more convenient to assess proteinuria and albuminuria levels using the ratio of protein or albumin to creatinine in an untimed ('spot') urine sample. Other markers of kidney damage include:

- Abnormalities in urine sediment (e.g. tubular cells or casts).
- Abnormal findings on imaging studies (e.g. hydronephrosis, asymmetry in kidney size, polycystic kidney disease, or small echogenic kidneys).

Table 3.1 Definitions of proteinuria and albuminuria

	Urine collection method	Normal	Microalbuminuria	Albuminuria or clinical proteinuria
Total protein	24h excretion (varies with method)	<300mg/day	NA	>300mg/day
	Spot urine dipstick	<30mg/dL	NA	>30mg/dL
	Spot urine protein-to-creatinine ratio (varies by method)	<200mg/g	NA	>200mg/g
Albumin	24h excretion	<30mg/day	30–300mg/day	>300mg/day
	Spot urine albumin-specific dipstick	<3mg/day	>3mg/day	NA
	Spot urine albumin-to-creatinine ratio (varies by gender)[a]	<17mg/g (men)	17–250mg/g (men)	>250mg/g (men)
		<25mg/g (women)	25–355mg/g (women)	>355mg/g (women)

[a] Gender-specific, cut-off values are from a single study. The use of the same cut-off value for men and women leads to higher prevalence rates for women than for men. Current recommendations from the American Diabetes Association define cut-off values for spot urine albumin-to-creatinine ratio for microalbuminuria and albuminuria as 30 and 300mg/g, respectively, without regard to gender; NA=not available. Used with permission from the National Kidney Foundation (NKF).

- Abnormalities in blood and urine chemistry measurements (e.g. renal tubular acidosis).
- History of transplantation.

Kidney function

Reduced kidney function is also defined as CKD. The level of GFR is usually accepted as the best overall index of level of kidney function in health and disease. A level lower than 60mL/min/1.73m^2 is defined as CKD.

Why is GFR less than 60mL/min/1.73m^2 defined as CKD?

- In young adults, the normal value for GFR is approximately 120–130mL/min/1.73m^2.
- Normal values vary according to age, sex, and body size.
- A GFR less than 60mL/min/1.73m^2 represents the loss of half or more of the adult level of normal kidney function and is associated with an increased prevalence of systemic complications.

How does GFR change with age?

- GFR declines with age by approximately 1mL/min/1.73m^2 per year after the third decade.
- More than 47% of individuals aged 70 years and older have estimated GFR less than 60mL/min/1.73m^2 and therefore, are defined as having CKD.
- Most elderly people with CKD have systemic diseases that cause kidney disease and therefore, the decreased kidney function is likely to truly reflect kidney disease. However, more research is required.
- Regardless of the cause, a GFR below 60mL/min/1.73m^2 in the elderly is an independent predictor of adverse outcomes such as death or CVD.

Many national and international organizations recommend the use of serum creatinine-based estimating equations as the primary assessment of kidney function in standard clinical practice. The Modification of Diet in Renal Disease (MDRD) study equation and Cockcroft–Gault equation provide useful estimates of GFR in adults. The MDRD study

The importance of accurate GFR estimates in the elderly

Decreased GFR is associated with an increased risk of a wide variety of other outcomes, including acute kidney injury and higher rates of medical errors in hospitalized patients.

The elderly have a high use of medications and therefore, the use of GFR for adjustment of drug doses is especially important in the elderly. Inaccurate estimates will lead to over- or under-dosage of medications.

equation is more accurate and precise than both the Cockcroft–Gault equation and measured creatinine clearance for persons with a GFR less than approximately 60mL/min/1.73m². There are strengths and limitations of all estimating equations and understanding them is important for optimal use.

- GFR estimating equations will not perform as well in populations and settings other than those in which they were developed. Both the MDRD study equation and Cockcroft–Gault equation would not work as well in the following populations:
  - Healthy populations.
  - Other racial, ethnic, or geographic groups.
  - In individuals in whom creatinine production would be expected to differ from the general population (e.g. extremes of body size, high levels of dietary meat intake, overweight or obesity, malnutrition, amputation, or conditions associated with muscle wasting).
  - Pregnant women.
- GFR estimating equations should be used in conjunction with the clinical context. For example, a persistent GFR less than 60mL/min/1.73m² is defined as CKD. Given the imprecision of the available GFR estimating equations, some people with estimated GFR just under 60mL/min/1.73m² will have a measured GFR that is greater than 60mL/min/1.73m². In these instances, a clinician must turn to alternative information such as the presence of kidney

damage or CKD risk factors to guide clinical decisions about the presence of CKD.

◆ GFR estimating equations cannot be used for patients not in the steady state.

Some studies suggest that GFR estimates based on cystatin C and creatinine together are more accurate than estimates based on creatinine alone. However, cystatin C-based GFR estimates are not more accurate than creatinine-based estimating equations. If an accurate estimate of GFR is required, a clearance measurement should be obtained using either a 24-hour urine collection for creatinine clearance or by measuring clearance of an exogenous filtration marker such as iothalamate or iohexol.

Classification of CKD

The severity of CKD is classified based on the level of GFR (Table 3.2). Lower GFR levels represent more advanced CKD stages and are associated with an increased risk for complications of CKD (see 'Complications of decreased kidney function'). Continued progression of CKD eventually leads to kidney failure, which is defined as an estimated GFR of less than $15mL/min/1.73m^2$ or the need for dialysis or kidney transplantation.

The stage of CKD is only one dimension for classification. CKD is a heterogeneous disease and the clinical course may vary considerably among patients. Other factors to consider in evaluating the severity of CKD are:

◆ The cause of CKD.

◆ The presence and severity of comorbid conditions.

◆ The rate of progression.

◆ The presence and severity of complications related to CKD.

Clinical action plan

The stage of CKD is linked to specific intervention guidelines (Table 3.2). The action plan includes recommended care for each stage as well as attention to the risks for progression to a more advanced stage. Three key points must be emphasized.

Table 3.2 NKF/Kidney Disease: Improving Global Outcomes (KDIGO) quality initiative classification and action plan for stages of CKD[†]

Stage	Description	GFR (mL/min/1.73m^2)	Prevalence*, n (%)	Actions
–	At increased risk and no kidney damage	≥60 (with chronic kidney disease risk factors)		Screening; chronic kidney disease, risk reduction
1	Kidney damage with normal or increased GFR	≥90	3,600,000 (1.8)	Diagnosis and treatment, treatment of comorbid conditions, slowing progression, CVD risk reduction
2	Kidney damage with mild decreased GFR	60–89	6,500,000 (3.2)	Estimating progression
3[‡]	Moderately decreased GFR	30–59	15,500,000 (7.7)	Evaluating and treating complications
4	Severely decreased GFR	15–29	700,000 (0.4)	Preparation for RRT
5	Kidney failure	<15 or dialysis	400,000 (0.2)	RRT (if patient wishes)

* Prevalence for CKD stage 5 is from the USRDS for people on treatment with dialysis or transplantation as well as an estimate of 0.36 untreated kidney failure patients for every treated patient. Prevalence for CKD stages 1–4 is projected from the NHANES (1999–2004) for the population of 200 million adults aged 20 years or older in 2000.

[†] NKF/KDOQI clinical practice guidelines for chronic kidney disease: evaluation, classification, and stratification. The action plan is cumulative in that each stage incorporates recommendations from the previous stage. Updated and reprinted with permission from National Kidney Foundation.

[‡] The National Institute for Health and Clinical Excellence (NICE) in the United Kingdom advocates splitting CKD Stage 3 into 2 categories: eGFR 30–44 and 45–59ml/min per 1.73m^2.

♦ The action plan is cumulative in that recommended care at each stage of disease includes care for less severe stages.

♦ The care for patients with CKD requires multiple interventions, and such providing appropriate care requires the coordinated multidisciplinary effort of primary care physicians (PCPs), allied health care workers, and other specialists in addition to nephrologists.

♦ The management of each stage of the disease must take into consideration CKD and CVD as well as other comorbid conditions. The stage-specific clinical action plan is a guide, not a replacement, for the physician's assessment of the needs of a specific patient.

Natural history and outcomes of CKD

What are the major outcomes of CKD?

+ Progressive loss of kidney function.

+ Complications of CKD.

+ CVD.

Rationale for a conceptual model, irrespective of aetiology

A conceptual model for the course of CKD is shown in Figure 3.1. This model describes the natural history of CKD, beginning with antecedent

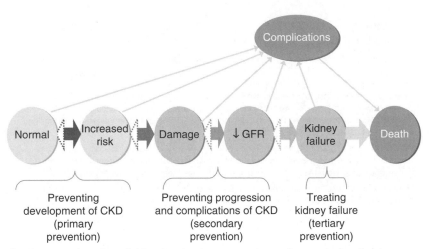

Fig. 3.1 Conceptual model for the development, progression, and complication of CKD

This diagram shows the continuum of development, progression, and complications of CKD. 'Complications' refer to all complications of CKD and its treatment, including complications of decreased GFR and CVD. Stages of prevention are shown along the continuum. The horizontal arrows pointing from left to right emphasize the progressive nature of CKD; however, the rate of progression is variable and not all patients progress. Interventions in earlier stages may slow or prevent the progression to later stages. The dashed arrowheads pointing from right to left signify that remission to earlier stages of kidney disease may be possible, but this is less frequent than progression. Reprinted with permission from Levey, et al., 2009 (modified and reprinted with permission from the National Kidney Foundation).

conditions, followed by the stages of CKD (kidney damage, decreased GFR, and kidney failure) and other associated outcomes.

Kidney disease tends to worsen over time by transitions through a defined sequence of stages, regardless of the underlying susceptibility to disease, the specific cause of kidney damage, or the rate of progression through each stage.

There is also a pathophysiological basis for describing the natural history of CKD, irrespective of aetiology.

A loss of functional nephrons leads to compensatory hypertrophy and hyperfiltration by the remaining nephrons as a mechanism to adapt to the loss of nephron mass. This seemingly adaptive process of hyperfiltration and hypertrophy eventually leads to maladaptive changes, including the development of proteinuria. Proteinuria, in turn, leads to tubular damage, interstitial inflammation, and nephrosclerosis, further reducing the nephron number and fuelling a self-perpetuating cycle of nephron destruction, culminating in uraemia. Animal and human studies both suggest that this pattern is similar across disease types. For example, it has been observed that even after the initial disease activity abates, a relentless progression to kidney failure often occurs, with a rate of GFR decline more characteristic of the specific individual rather than the specific aetiology of the kidney disease.

Rate of progression

Kidney failure is the most visible outcome of CKD, yet relatively few patients with CKD develop kidney failure. The rate of progression through the stages depends upon:

- The stage of CKD.
- The presence of risk factors for progression (see below for the listing of risk factors).

The rate of progression is highly variable. For example, if the rate of decline is 4mL/min/1.73m^2 per year, then the interval from a GFR of 60mL/min/1.73m^2 to the onset of kidney failure (defined by GFR <15mL/min/1.73m^2) would be 11 to 12 years. This rate of decline is considered fast. By contrast, if the rate of decline in GFR is 1mL/min/1.73m^2 per year, an elderly individual with a GFR of 60mL/min/1.73m^2 may not reach kidney failure in his or her lifetime. Thus, older patients, patients with a higher GFR, and those with few risk factors may not develop kidney failure in their lifetime. Some patients may not have any observable progression. Recent studies have demonstrated that older patients with CKD are more likely to die than progress to kidney failure.

Complications of decreased kidney function

The systemic complications of decreased GFR are those that make up the uraemic syndrome associated with kidney failure. They can begin at levels well above those associated with kidney failure (Figure 3.2). Complications of CKD include:

- Hypertension.
- Anaemia.
- Malnutrition.
- Bone and mineral disorders.
- Neuropathy.
- Decreased quality of life.
- Poor sleep.
- Fatigue.
- CVD.
- An increased risk for complications of care such as medication and medical errors, and perioperative complications.

The impact of CKD on other comorbid conditions, such as infectious diseases or malignancies, is also considerable.

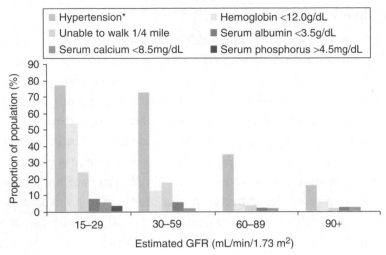

Fig. 3.2 Estimated prevalence of complications related to CKD according to the eGFR in the general population

Hypertension was defined as a systolic pressure of 140mmHg or higher, or a diastolic pressure of 90mmHg or higher, or the receipt of anti-hypertensive medication. The study population includes participants in the third National Health and Nutrition Evaluation Survey (1988–1994) who were 20 years of age or older. A total of 10,162 participants with a mean age of 39 years had a GFR greater than 90mL/min/1.73m2; 4,404 with a mean age of 54 years had a GFR of 60–89; 961 with a mean age of 72 years had a GFR of 30–59; and 52 with a mean age of 75 years had a GFR of 15–29. Adapted from National Kidney Foundation.

What are examples of medication errors that can occur if a physician fails to recognize CKD and the level of kidney function?

- The level of kidney function is important for the selection of appropriate medications and doses for all conditions.

- Errors in dose increase the risk for drug-drug interactions, adverse drug reactions, complications of routine procedures, hospitalizations, and death.

- Anti-inflammatory agents are especially important because they are widely used in the elderly, but are contraindicated with CKD and may be an important cause of an acute decline in GFR in the elderly.

- Oral phosphate-based bowel preparations have recently been associated with development of decline in GFR.

Cardiovascular disease

Chapter 6 discusses CVD and CKD extensively. CVD is the primary cause of death in patients with CKD. Irrespective of age, sex, race, and the presence of diabetes, rates of CVD-related mortality are 10 to 20 times higher in dialysis patients compared to the general population. Decreased GFR and albuminuria are powerful risk factors for CVD morbidity and mortality in population-based studies. The independent association of CKD and adverse CVD outcomes may be associated with an increased level of non-traditional CVD risk factors or undiagnosed vascular disease or alternatively, an indicator for the severity of diagnosed vascular disease. As described below, CVD is a risk factor for CKD that is treatable and potentially preventable.

How does CKD affect the diagnosis and management of CVD and its risk factors?

- Diagnostic test selection and interpretation differ in CKD. Cardiac enzymes are retained at decreased GFR, reducing their specificity for acute coronary syndromes. Furthermore, iodinated contrast agents used in cardiac imaging procedures present an increased risk to the kidney due to their toxicity and gadolinium's toxicity to the skin and connective tissue.

- The management of CVD risk factor conditions such as diabetes and hypertension differs among patients with and without CKD.

- Thiazide-type diuretics are recommended for elderly patients with hypertension and CVD risk factors, but angiotensin-converting enzyme inhibitors (ACEi) or angiotensin receptor blockers (ARB) are preferred for patients with albuminuria.

Risk factors for CKD

In this section, we define the different types of risk factors for CKD, including conditions that increase risk for the development of kidney disease as well as risk factors that increase the risk of progression and complications associated with CKD (Table 3.3). These factors commonly represent a continuum of events as there is often overlap between the different types of factors.

Table 3.3 Risk factors for the development, progression, and complications of CKD

Risk factor	Definition	Examples
Development	Increases susceptibility to kidney damage	Older age, family history of CKD, US racial or ethnic minority status, low income, reduced kidney mass, hyperfiltration states
	Directly initiates kidney damage	Diabetes, high blood pressure, obesity, dyslipidaemia, autoimmune diseases, infections, stones, obstruction, neoplasia, recovery from acute injury
Progression	Worsens kidney damage or accelerates GFR decline	Higher level of proteinuria
	Increases the risk for complications of decreased GFR	Factors related to hypertension, anaemia, malnutrition, bone and mineral disorders, neuropathy, drugs and procedures with kidney or systemic toxicity
Complications	Accelerate the onset or recurrence of CVD	Traditional CVD risk factors, non-traditional 'CKD-related' risk factors
	Increase morbidity and mortality in kidney failure	Late referral, dialysis factors, comorbid conditions

Types of risk factors

Development factors

Development factors that increase one's risk for kidney disease can be divided into susceptibility and initiation factors. Individuals with susceptibility or initiation factors are at increased risk for CKD and should be tested for CKD.

What are susceptibility factors?

Susceptibility factors are characteristics that put an individual at risk of developing kidney damage when exposed to an initiation factor.

◆ Genetic or developmental: low birthweight and intrauterine growth retardation resulting in reduced nephron mass.

◆ Demographic characteristics: age, race, ethnicity, or socio-economic status also place individuals at an increased risk for the development of kidney damage.

Susceptibility factors may explain why a family history of kidney disease, regardless of the cause, places an individual at an increased risk for the development of kidney disease.

What are initiation factors?

Initiation factors are conditions that can directly cause kidney damage.

- Diabetes.
- High blood pressure.
- Obstructive uropathy.
- Drug toxicity.
- Urinary tract infections.
- Immune-mediated mechanisms.
- Direct drug toxicity.

Exposure to initiating conditions, together with the presence of susceptibility factors, determines whether or not an individual develops kidney damage.

Progression factors

Progression factors worsen kidney damage and lead to further decline in kidney function. Kidney disease may progress because the disorder responsible for the inciting damage is continuous or as a result of pathways independent of the initial damage. Progression factors influence the risk for and rate of decline in kidney function.

- Traditional progression factors:
  - Elevated blood pressure.
  - Higher level of proteinuria.
  - Poor glycaemic control in diabetes.
  - Ongoing drug toxicity and smoking.
- Non-traditional risk factors are now being recognized and may include:
  - Elevated asymmetric dimethylarginine.
  - C-reactive protein.
  - Soluble tumour necrosis factor (TNF) receptor 2
  - Apolipoprotein A-IV.

Complications

- Increase risk for complications of decreased GFR (see section on complications of decreased kidney function).

- Accelerate onset or recurrence of CVD (see Chapter 6).
- Increase morbidity and mortality in kidney failure:
  - Adequacy of dialysis.
  - Type of vascular access.
  - Compliance with dialysis prescription.
  - Nutritional status.
  - Presence of CVD.

What is the relationship between CKD and family history?

- CKD aggregates in families.
- Some kidney diseases are inherited, e.g. polycystic kidney disease and Alport's nephropathy.
- There is an increased risk for the development of kidney disease in first-degree relatives of patients with kidney failure, even for diseases that are not thought to be inherited.
  - In a cohort of incident dialysis patients, 20% reported a family history of kidney failure among first- or second- degree relatives.
  - Another study demonstrated that having two or more first-degree relatives with kidney disease has been shown to be associated with a 10-fold increase in the odds of kidney failure.
  - More recently, the level of estimated GFR has been shown to be heritable.

What are some genes that have been identified as being involved in kidney disease?

Recent data on the role of genetics in the development of kidney provide some explanation for the aggregation of kidney disease in families.

- Angiotensin-converting enzyme (ACE) and angiotensin gene polymorphisms have been associated with:
  - An increased susceptibility or initiation of CKD for kidney diseases of diverse aetiologies such as Henoch–Schönlein purpura, diabetic nephropathy, and hypertension.
  - The progression of kidney disease in patients with established disease.

- The e2 allele of the apolipoprotein E (APOE) gene was shown to be associated with faster progression compared to the e4 allele.
- Single nucleotide polymorphism in the gene MTHFS was associated with CKD in both the Framingham Heart Study and white participants of the Atherosclerosis Risk In Communities (ARIC) study.
  - The MTHFS gene codes for the enzyme methenyltetrahydrofolate synthetase which has been reported in play a role in folate turnover and accumulation.
  - The mechanism by which abnormalities in this enzyme could lead to susceptibility, initiation, or progression of kidney disease is not known at this time.

It is likely that the next decade will lead to further understanding of the role of specific genes in the susceptibility to, initiation and progression of kidney disease.

How does race and socio-economic factors affect the prevalence of CKD?

Effects of race on CKD

- Racial and ethnic minorities have a higher prevalence of CKD.
- Blacks are reported to progress faster than whites, which may account for their development of kidney failure at an earlier age than whites, even after adjusting for diabetes and hypertension.
- While the rates of CKD progression are not as well understood for other racial groups, it is known that the incidence rates for kidney failure are higher.
- The reasons for these differences are not known and may be related to environmental or genetic factors.

Effects of socio-economic status on CKD

- Socio-economic differences create barriers to achieving optimal health through the following factors:
  - Decreased birth rates.
  - Decreased access to health care.
  - Late referral to nephrologists.

- Poor nutrition.

- Increased exposure to environmental nephrotoxins.

• An increased risk for the development of chronic diseases such as obesity, diabetes, and hypertension:

   - Leads to an increase in risk factors for the development of CKD.

   - Suboptimal care of these conditions would then lead to a faster progression of CKD. Comparisons of same racial and ethnic groups showed that populations of lower socio-economic status had a faster progressive CKD than populations with higher socio-economic status. The trend persisted after adjustment for health awareness, health care access, and behavioural and physiological factors.

Evidence for the role of genetics in the racial difference in CKD prevalence

A recent study showed that even though racial disparity in ESRD incidence was more pronounced in poorer neighbourhoods, disparities persisted, even in the least impoverished neighbourhoods.

In addition, there are certainly biologic differences among races.

• For example, hypovitaminosis D levels have been shown to be higher in blacks.

   - Higher levels are associated with hypertension and diabetes as well as inflammation and fibrosis, which would all lead to faster progression.

• Blacks have higher rates of sickle cell trait, which may contribute to the development and faster progression of CKD.

Together, these data suggest that the racial differences in CKD development and progression are due to both environmental and genetics factors, which can also influence each other.

What is the relationship between CVD and CKD?

The relationship between CKD and CVD is complex (see Chapter 6). It is well recognized that CKD is a risk factor for CVD.

• The leading cause of mortality in patients with CKD is CVD.

- ♦ CVD may also be a risk factor for the development and progression of CKD.

- ♦ A high prevalence of shared traditional risk factors for CVD such as diabetes and hypertension may provide one explanation for the high prevalence of CKD in patients with CVD as well as the converse.

- ♦ Certain characteristics of patients with CVD predispose them to the development of CKD such as:

  - Hypoperfusion.

  - High atherosclerotic burden.

  - Renal vascular disease.

  - Hypertension.

  - Specific diagnostic procedures that may involve radiocontrast dye exposure or atheroemboli.

- ♦ It has been suggested that inadequate treatment or therapeutic nihilism by both cardiologists and nephrologists caring for patients with an established kidney or cardiac disease may be another potential reason for this association and for worse outcomes for CVD in patients with CKD and faster progression of CKD.

References

Bricker, N.S., Morrin, P.A., Kime, S.W. Jr., 1960. The pathologic physiology of chronic Bright's disease. An exposition of the 'intact nephron hypothesis'. *American Journal of Medicine*, 28, pp.77–98.

Chan, M.R., Dall, A.T., Fletcher, K.E., Lu, N., Trivedi, H., 2007. Outcomes in patients with chronic kidney disease referred late to nephrologists: a meta-analysis. *American Journal of Medicine*, 120(12), pp.1063–70.

Coresh, J., Selvin, E., Stevens, L.A., Manzi, J., Kusek, J.W., Eggers, P., Van Lente, F., Levey, A.S., 2007. Prevalence of Chronic Kidney Disease in the United States. *Journal of the American Medical Association*, 298(17), pp.2038–47.

Fried, L., Solomon, C., Shlipak, M., Seliger, S., Stehman–Breen, C., Bleyer, A., Chaves, P., Furberg, C., Kuller, L., Newman, A., 2004. Inflammatory and Prothrombotic Markers and the Progression of Renal Disease in Elderly Individuals. *Journal of the American Society of Nephrology*, 15(12), pp.3184–91.

Hsu, C.Y., Ordonez, J.D., Chertow, G.M., Fan, D., McCulloch, C.E., Go, A.S., 2008. The risk of acute renal failure in patients with chronic kidney disease. *Kidney International*, 74(1), pp.101–7.

Imai, E., Matsuo, S., 2008. Chronic kidney disease in Asia. *Lancet*, 371(9631), pp.2147–8.

Keijzer–Veen, M.G., Schrevel, M., Finken, M.J., Dekker, F.W., Nauta, J., Hille, E.T., Frolich, M., van der Heijden, B.J.; Dutch POPS-19 Collaborative Study Group, 2005. Microalbuminuria and lower glomerular filtration rate at young adult age in subjects born very premature and after intrauterine growth retardation. *Journal of the American Society of Nephrology*, 16(9), pp.2762–8.

Khurana, A., McLean, L., Atkinson, S., Foulks, C.J., 2008. The effect of oral sodium phosphate drug products on renal function in adults undergoing bowel endoscopy. *Archives of Internal Medicine*, 168(6), pp.593–7.

Lei, H.H., Perneger, T.V., Klag, M.J., Whelton, P.K., Coresh, J., 1998. Familial aggregation of renal disease in a population-based case-control study. *Journal of the American Society of Nephrology*, 9(7), pp.1270–6.

Levey, A.S., Eckardt, K.U., Tsukamoto, Y., Levin, A., Coresh, J., Rossert, J., De Zeeuw, D., Hostetter, T.H., Lameire, N., Eknoyan, G., 2005. Definition and classification of chronic kidney disease: A position statement from Kidney Disease: Improving Global Outcomes (KDIGO). *Kidney International*, 67(6), pp.2089–100.

Levey, A.S., Stevens, L.A., Coresh, J., 2009. Conceptual model of CKD: applications and implications. *American Journal of Kidney Diseases*, 53(3 Suppl 3), S4–16.

Levin, A., Djurdjev, O., Barrett, B., Burgess, E., Carlisle, E., Ethier, J., Jindal, K., Mendelssohn, D., Tobe, S., Singer, J., Thompson, C., 2001. Cardiovascular disease in patients with chronic kidney disease: Getting to the heart of the matter. *American Journal of Kidney Diseases*, 38(6), 1398–407.

Powe, N.R., 2008. Let's get serious about racial and ethnic disparities. *Journal of the American Society of Nephrology*, 19(7), pp.1271–5.

Sarnak, M.J., Levey, A.S., Schoolwerth, A.C., Coresh, J., Culleton, B., Hamm, L.L., McCullough, P.A., Kasiske, B.L., Kelepouris, E., Klag, M.J., Parfrey, P., Pfeffer, M., Raij, L., Spinosa, D.J., Wilson, P.W.; American Heart Association Councils on Kidney in Cardiovascular Disease, High Blood Pressure Research, Clinical Cardiology, and Epidemiology and Prevention, 2003. Kidney disease as a risk factor for development of cardiovascular disease: A statement from the American Heart Association Councils on Kidney in Cardiovascular Disease, High Blood Pressure Research, Clinical Cardiology, and Epidemiology and Prevention. *Hypertension*, 42(5), pp.1050–65.

Shlipak, M.G., Sarnak, M.J., Katz, R., Fried, L.F., Seliger, S.L., Newman, A.B., Siscovick, D.S., Stehman–Breen, C., 2005. Cystatin C and the risk of death and cardiovascular events among elderly persons. *New England Journal of Medicine*, 352(20), 2049–60.

Singh, G.R., Hoy, W.E., 2004. Kidney volume, blood pressure, and albuminuria: findings in an Australian aboriginal community. *American Journal of Kidney Diseases*, 43(2), pp.254–9.

Steinman, M.A., Landefeld, C.S., Rosenthal, G.E., Berthenthal, D., Sen, S., Kabol, P.J., 2006. Polypharmacy and prescribing quality in older people. *Journal of the American Geriatric Society*, 54(10), pp.16–23.

Stevens, L.A., Coresh, J., Deysher, A.E., Feldman, H.I., Lash, J.P., Nelson, R., Rahman, M., Deysher, A.E., Zhang, Y.L., Schmid, C.H., Levey, A.S., 2007. Evaluation of the MDRD Study equation in a large diverse population. *Journal of the American Society of Nephrology*, 18(10), pp.2749–57.

Stevens, L.A., Coresh, J., Greene, T., Levey, A.S., 2006. Assessing kidney function - measured and estimated glomerular filtration rate. *New England Journal of Medicine*, 354(23), pp.2473–83.

Stevens, L.A., Coresh, J., Schmid, C.H., Feldman, H.I., Froissart, M., Kusek, J., Rossert, J., Van Lente, F, Bruce, R.D. 3rd, Zhang, Y.L., Greene, T., Levey, A.S., 2008. Estimating GFR using serum cystatin C alone and in combination with serum creatinine: a pooled analysis of 3,418 individuals with CKD. *American Journal of Kidney Diseases*, 51(3), pp.395–406.

Chapter 4

Recommendations for screening and detection of chronic kidney disease

Bisher Kawar and Meguid El Nahas

Introduction

Worldwide, CKD is increasingly becoming a major health care issue. This is seen both as a rise in the number of patients reaching end-stage renal disease (ESRD), requiring renal replacement therapy (RRT; dialysis or transplantation), and a perceived rise in the prevalence of earlier stages of CKD. This chapter explores various aspects of screening for CKD.

The basic principles for establishing a screening programme have been described by Wilson and Jungner in 1968 (Wilson & Jungner, 1968). Those principles are summarized in Table 4.1. The first part of this chapter discusses whether CKD satisfies those criteria to justify screening. The second part provides a practical guide to screening, highlighting potential groups where screening is most warranted and summarizing current screening recommendations.

Principles of screening and CKD

Screening criterion 1: the condition sought should be an important health problem

CKD detection is rising worldwide. Estimates of CKD prevalence vary according to the definition of CKD. Adopting the US National Kidney Foundation (NKF)/Kidney Disease Outcomes Quality Initiative

Table 4.1 Wilson–Jungner screening criteria: their applicability to CKD

Criterion	Applicability and evidence
The condition being screened for should be an important health problem.	Yes (evidence)
The natural history of the condition should be well understood.	No
There should be a detectable, early stage.	Yes (consensus)
Treatment at an early stage should be of more benefit than at a later stage.	Yes: Proteinuria (evidence) BP (evidence) CVD risk modification (consensus)
A suitable test for the early stage, which is available and acceptable.	Yes
Intervals for repeating the test should be determined.	Opinion-based
Adequate health service provision should be made for the extra clinical workload resulting from screening.	Country-based
The risks, both physical and psychological, should be less than the benefits.	Yes, when screening is targeted

(KDOQI) classification (KDOQI, 2002), the third National Health and Examination Survey (NHANES III) estimated a prevalence of 11% in the US (Coresh, et al., 2007). However, this includes those with CKD stages 1 and 2. The prevalence of CKD stage 3 and above (eGFR <60mL/min/1.73m^2) is 4.7%, of whom only 0.2% having CKD stage 5 (ESRD). In Europe, a recent study from Norway showed a similar prevalence of CKD 3 (Hallan, et al., 2006). Data from the Netherlands suggested that around 7% may have microalbuminuria (MA). Data from the developing world are sparse, but surveys in China suggest that around 2–3% of the general population may have CKD (Chen, et al., 2005).

It is important to be aware of the limitations of such CKD prevalence surveys as they depend to a large extent on the validity of the screening methods applied. Many have relied on the detection of MA which, as will be discussed below, is anything but specific for CKD. Others relied on formulae-based calculations of GFR, with the MDRD formula being the most commonly used. The latter may prove inadequate for estimating GFR in the general population and individuals with GFR within the normal range. Most studies relied on single, cross-sectional analysis and seldom confirmed the chronic nature of the detected abnormalities. With that in mind, the true prevalence of progressive CKD remains unknown.

Cardiovascular disease (CVD) mortality is the main cause of chronic, non-communicable disease death worldwide; in excess of 20 millions die every year from CVD. CKD is likely to impact on the burden of CVD morbidity and mortality and adversely affect the outcome of patients with diabetes and hypertension. This is also the case of MA which is increasingly recognized as a useful CVD risk marker. CKD patients have high rates of cardiovascular mortality and morbidity (Go, et al., 2004; Henry, et al., 2002). One study showed an independent graded increase in the relative risk (RR) of cardiovascular mortality from 1.2 in patients with GFR 45–59mL/min/1.73m^2, rising to 5.9 in those with GFR <15mL/min/1.73m^2 (Go, et al., 2004). In fact, the majority of CKD patients are likely to die from CVD before they reach ESRD. The increased cardiovascular risk in CKD is multifactorial and includes anaemia and hypertension, but also chronic inflammation and changes in calcium/phosphate homeostasis. The association between CKD and CVD is likely to magnify the importance of the former in terms of health care cost. This may prove to be one of the major cost implications of CKD.

The cost burden of ESRD is enormous. In the US, the expected expenditure on ESRD is expected to exceed US$ 28 million by 2010 (USRDS, 2003). In Europe, RRT takes up to 2% of health care budget with <0.1% of the population requiring treatment (Lameire, et al., 2005). It is noteworthy that worldwide, 90% of patients receiving dialysis treatment are in developed countries, which means that there is a much higher hidden global burden of ESRD. It also implies that ESRD in the developing world is an unmet health care challenge and a death sentence due to the unavailability or inability to afford RRT.

Screening criterion 2: there should be a detectable pre-clinical stage and there should be a suitable test that is acceptable to the population

There are some clear markers of CKD that are either urine-based (MA, proteinuria, haematuria) or serum-based (creatinine-based GFR estimation). Rarely, ultrasound screening is indicated, e.g. relatives of patients with cystic kidney disease. The screening tests are discussed below.

Microalbuminuria (MA)

MA was first described in diabetic patients as urine albumin excretion (UAE) below the level of detection by conventional dipstick (Viberti, et al., 1982), which was later recognized to be predictive of overt diabetic nephropathy (Mogensen, 1984).

MA is now defined as UAE of 20–200µg/min, which equates to around 30–300mg of albumin in 24 hours. This is estimated by measuring albumin-to-creatinine ratio (ACR). The current definition of MA in terms of ACR is 2.5–30mg/mmol for males and 3.5–30mg/mmol for females. The reason for the difference is that creatinine excretion is lower in females due to lower muscle mass.

The presence of MA has to be confirmed in at least two samples of three due to intra-individual variation in UAE of 40–60% in one study (Dyer, et al., 2004).

The significance of MA in predicting CKD comes from studies on patients with diabetes mellitus. The earliest evidence that MA predicts overt nephropathy and progressive kidney disease came from patients with type 1 diabetes mellitus (Viberti, et al., 1982). Similar evidence from patients with type 2 diabetes mellitus shortly followed (Mogensen, 1984).

In the general population, the evidence that MA predicts CKD is less clear-cut. Cross-sectional data suggest that up to 7% of the population may have MA (Hillege, et al., 2002). However, the majority of patients with renal insufficiency (GFR <60mL/min/1.73m^2) do not have MA. Data from NHANES III suggest that 63% of patients with GFR <30 do not have MA (Garg, et al., 2002). Similarly, a Japanese study showed that only 17% of subjects with GFR <60mL/min have MA (Konta, et al., 2006).

There is lack of prospective data on the renal prognosis of raised UAE in non-diabetics. One study from the Prevention of Renal and Vascular End Stage Disease (PREVEND) group, including 6,022 participants with over-representation of microalbuminuric subjects, found that the risk of developing renal impairment (eGFR <60mL/min/1.73m^2)

increases with increasing UAE (Verhave, et al., 2004). However, this study included a significant percentage of diabetics and hypertensives. The PREVEND study also confirmed the variable and reversible nature of MA as obese individuals who lost weight demonstrated regression of MA.

On balance, apart from patients with diabetes, there is no evidence that MA is a good screening test for CKD.

However, MA is a strong predictor of CVD in both the diabetic and the general population (Amlov, et al., 2005; Borch–Johnsen, et al., 1999; Dinncen, et al., 1997; Hillege, et al., 2002; Romundstad, et al., 2003; Yudkin, et al., 1988; Yuyun, et al., 2004). Hence, in the context of screening for CVD in patients with CKD, MA may be an additional useful screening tool in non-diabetics. Whether it adds much in terms of prognosis to current predictors such as anaemia, hypertension, dyslipidaemia, and smoking remains to be determined.

Proteinuria

Proteinuria is a marker of CKD and a predictor of its progression. Several studies have identified proteinuria as a powerful predictor of ESRD (Iseki, et al., 1996; Klahr, et al., 1994). Therefore, screening for proteinuria could potentially identify those at highest risk of progressive CKD/ESRD.

The tests

Urine dipstick Urine dipstick has a sensitivity and specificity for detecting urinary protein levels >200mg/L of the order 80–95%, depending on the specific product (Craig, et al., 2002; Siedner, et al., 2008). Albumin-specific dipstick provides better specificity. Causes for false positive and false negative results are summarized in Table 4.2.

Total protein This is an easy and relatively cheap test that detects protein at a concentration of >100–200mg/L. It is not specific to albumin and is insensitive to positively charged proteins such as immunoglobulins. A persistently positive (on two or more occasions) should be followed by quantification (see below).

Albuminuria Dipstick tests that are specific for albumin are also available. Those are particularly useful when screening for microalbuminuria.

Quantification Studies have shown that the outcome of CKD relates to the degree of proteinuria usually expressed as daily protein excretion.

Table 4.2 Protein dipstick: causes of false readings

Causes of false positive	Causes of false negative
Heavily alkaline urine (pH >8)	Positively charged proteins, e.g. tubular proteins, Bence–Jones protein
Dehydration causing increased concentration	Excessive hydration causing low concentration
Transient increase in urinary protein excretion: exercise, infection	
Haematuria	
Drugs, e.g. penicillin, cephalosporins, miconazole, contrast medium	

Furthermore, evidence suggests that a reduction of proteinuria with renin-angiotensin-aldosterone system (RAAS) inhibiting drugs is only beneficial when the protein excretion is >1g/24h (Jafar, et al., 2001). Similarly, intensive blood pressure treatment to a target mean arterial pressure (MAP) <92mmHg (<130/80mmHg) *vs* the conventional target of 107mmHg (<140/90) may be advantageous when proteinuria exceeds 1g/24h (Lea, et al., 2005). Therefore, once proteinuria is detected on dipstick, it should be quantified by one of the following methods:

24h urine collection Although traditionally regarded as the gold standard, 24h collections are inconvenient to the patients and are often incomplete, leading to inaccurate results.

Timed overnight collection This may be easier to collect than 24h urine, but still poses a significant source of error due to inaccurate collections.

Spot urine protein-to-creatinine ratio (PCR) This is becoming the standard method for quantifying urine protein excretion. A PCR of 100mg/mmol is equivalent to about 1g of protein in 24h. Urine protein concentration can be affected by hydration status, e.g. dehydration leads to urinary concentration and hence, higher protein concentration. As creatinine excretion is constant under steady state conditions, correction for creatinine concentration would overcome the hydration effect.

Samples can be random or early morning. Early morning samples are preferable as they give a better indication of protein excretion without being influenced by, e.g. exercise or diet. They correlate better with 24-hour excretion and this has been shown in several studies (Marshall, 1991).

Spot urine ACR This has the same principle as PCR, but is more specific for albumin. Therefore, it is more appropriate when testing for MA or when other proteins such as immunoglobulin light chains are present in the urine.

The use of a quantitative method such as PCR as a primary screening method as opposed to preliminary screening with dipstick method

Table 4.3 Renal causes of isolated haematuria

Glomerulonephritis, e.g. IgA nephropathy
Hereditary nephritis, e.g. Alport's disease
Benign familial haematuria
Thin basement membrane disease

improves the sensitivity and specificity, but they are more costly (Craig, et al., 2002).

Haematuria

Haematuria is another manifestation of CKD. Some kidney diseases may present as isolated haematuria. Some examples are summarized in Table 4.3. Co-existence with proteinuria is highly suggestive of glomerular disease.

However, isolated haematuria may indicate a urological problem such as renal stone disease. In the elderly, it is imperative to rule out a urinary tract malignancy. Current guidelines suggest initial urological investigations in any patient presenting with isolated haematuria over the age of 50 years. In the developing world, isolated haematuria should trigger alarm bells for chronic infections such as schistosomiasis and urinary tract tuberculosis.

As with proteinuria, microscopic non-visible haematuria should be confirmed on two separate occasions in the absence of urinary infections. Confirmation of red cells on urine microscopy is also recommended.

Table 4.4 summarizes the causes of false positive and false negative results.

As a screening test for CKD, screening for haematuria does not substitute screening for proteinuria. Kidney disease presenting with

Table 4.4 Dipstick haematuria: causes of false readings

Causes of false positive	Causes of false negative
Myoglobin	High concentration of urinary ascorbic acid
Bacterial overgrowth	High nitrite concentration
	High urine density

isolated haematuria (absence of proteinuria and normal renal excretory function) usually have a good prognosis and therefore, the value of screening for isolated haematuria to detect kidney disease and prevent/ reduce morbidity or mortality is questionable.

Estimated GFR (eGFR)

The measurement of serum creatinine has been used for estimating renal function for a long time, despite well-known limitations. Those limitations include the effect of muscle mass which varies with age, dietary protein intake, and tubular secretion. Therefore, formulae have been derived to give a better estimate of renal function than serum creatinine alone. The Cockroft–Gault formula (Cockroft & Gault, 1976) has now been largely replaced by the MDRD formula (Levey, et al., 1999), which is the basis of the KDOQI classification of CKD (Table 4.5). The latter, in its most commonly used form, corrects for age, gender, and race (black race).

Table 4.5 KDOQI classification of CKD

Stage	Description
1	Kidney damage with normal kidney function (eGFR >90mL/min/1.73m^2)
2	Kidney damage with eGFR 60–89mL/min/1.73m^2
3	eGFR 30–59mL/min/1.73m^2
4	eGFR 16–29mL/min/1.73m^2
5	eGFR <15mL/min/1.73m^2

The use of eGFR as a screening tool is limited by the following factors:

- It is more expensive than urinary screening tests, especially when mass population screening is considered.

- The formula has not been validated in non-white, non-black individuals. The original MDRD equation was not validated in normal kidney function, diabetics (type 1), pregnancy, morbid obesity (BMI >40kg/m^2), and kidney transplant recipients (Levey, et al., 1999).

- The formula is not accurate in estimating GFR above 60mL/min/1.73m^2 (Froissart, et al., 2005).

- In the elderly population, in the absence of other manifestation of CKD such as proteinuria or hypertension, whether reduced GFR in the range of 45–60mL/min/1.73m^2 alone constitutes CKD is questionable. In fact, one study showed that the positive predictive value of GFR <60 for the presence of ≥1 CKD metabolic complication (abnormal potassium, phosphate, parathyroid hormone (PTH), haemoglobin, or bicarbonate) is only 34%, suggesting that some of those patients do not actually have CKD (Foley, et al., 2008). This can give rise to one of the major drawbacks of screening programmes, which is labelling non-diseased individuals as having a chronic disease, causing unnecessary anxiety.

In short, the sensitivity and specificity of eGFR as a screening test for CKD are not known. Therefore, mass population screening for CKD using GFR is not justified and run the risk of over-inflating the number of those with 'so-called CKD'. GFR should be reserved for screening high-risk groups such as diabetics, hypertensives, or those with other markers of kidney damage.

Screening criterion 3: there should be an acceptable treatment for patients with recognized disease

Interventions that affect the course of CKD and reduce the risk of ESRD

BP control Treatment of hypertension has been shown to reduce the progression of CKD, especially in proteinuric patients. Locatelli et al. (1996) showed that renal survival is significantly better in patients with MAP <107mmHg than those with higher BP. Interventional studies also showed that the rate of decline in renal function is faster in those with higher BP, but the effect is most marked in those with more than 1g proteinuria in 24 hours (Peterson, et al., 1995).

In patients with significant proteinuria (>1g/24h; PCR >100mg/mmol), ACEi/ARB agents are recommended as first-line treatment as a reduction of proteinuria is associated with better renal outcomes. This was shown in several studies such as the Ramipril Efficacy in Nephropathy (REIN) study and the African American Study of Kidney disease and hypertension (AASK) (Lea, et al., 2005) in non-diabetic CKD as well as the RENAAL and Irbesartan in Diabetic Nephropathy Trial (IDNT) studies in diabetic nephropathy (Atkins, et al., 2005).

In patients with non-proteinuric (<1g/24h) CKD, the control of hypertension should follow national guidelines, including, as in the UK guidelines, the use of calcium antagonists and diuretics as first-line therapy in view of the cost-effectiveness and good risk/benefit profile of this combination therapy.

Interventions that reduce CKD mortality/morbidity

CKD is associated with an increased risk of CVD (Go, et al., 2004; Henry, et al., 2002). In fact, it is likely that CKD patients with an eGFR <45mL/min are at the highest CVD risk with 25% incidence of events over a 10-year period. As well as reducing the risk of ESRD, an early identification of CKD should prompt aggressive management of cardiovascular risk factors such as hyperlipidaemia and smoking in order to the reduce the CKD-associated CVD. A recent meta-analysis suggests that statin therapy reduces CVD mortality in CKD, irrespective of stage (Strippoli, et al., 2008).

In addition to the classical cardiovascular risk factors, other CKD-specific factors can be addressed and treated such as anaemia and the so-called CKD-mineral bone disorder (CKD-MBD) which causes vascular calcification and accelerates atherosclerosis.

Furthermore, for those who progress to ESRD, an earlier identification is associated with better dialysis outcomes (Stack, 2003).

Screening criterion 4: the natural history of the disease is understood

The natural history of CKD is complex and not well understood. There may be several reasons for that. Firstly, CKD comprises a heterogeneous group of disorders, ranging from structural to glomerular to tubular diseases. There is evidence that the prognosis of CKD depends on the underlying disorder (Locatelli, et al., 1996). Secondly, the majority of CKD patients do not progress to ESRD. This is apparent from prevalence data where, e.g. in the US, the prevalence of CKD stage 3 is 4.3% compared to the prevalence of stage 5 at only 0.2%. The difference is due to the fact that the majority of CKD patients die from CVD before reaching ESRD and the fact that some cases of CKD do not progress. This discrepancy may have been compounded by the fact that labelling of elderly individuals with reduced GFR as 'CKD stage 3' generates a large pool of individuals with reduced, but stable renal function, who die of old age or the associated CVD.

Screening criterion 5: the cost of case-finding should be balanced with medical care availability

So far, we have established that CKD, by and large, satisfies most of the Wilson–Jungner criteria for screening, although there are many unanswered questions:

- CKD is an important health problem, but its true extent remains unknown.
- A pre-clinical stage of MA/proteinuria/haematuria or reduced GFR exists, but its predictive value for CKD awaits confirmation.
- There are acceptable screening tests with reasonable specificity and sensitivity despite the limitations discussed.

- There are treatments that alter the course of the disease and reduce the associated mortality/morbidity burden in spite of the fact that the natural history is not fully understood.

Therefore, the next question is whether screening will be cost-effective. To a large extent, this depends on the available healthcare resources and the health economic priorities. Those are understandably different between the developed and the developing worlds.

One study from the US showed that the cost per quality-adjusted-life year (QALY) of annual screening for proteinuria over the age of 50 years and treating with ACEi/ARB is US$ 282,818 (Boulware, et al., 2003). However, targeting hypertensives reduces the cost dramatically to US$ 18,621. This analysis did not take into consideration the impact of CKD detection on CVD morbidity and mortality.

Therefore, emphasis should shift towards screening higher risk groups. Those are discussed below in 'Targeted screening: high-risk groups'. Examples of screening programmes in the developing world such as India highlighted the cost-effectiveness of interventions targeting those with diabetes and hypertension with associated CKD. Better control of hypertension and diabetes, with presumably better outcomes, was achieved at a very low cost (Datta & Mani, 2006).

Targeted screening: high-risk groups

People with diabetes

All diabetics should be periodically screened for MA, according to most guidelines (UK CKD, ADA, KDOQI, UK NICE). MA is a marker of incipient nephropathy, but more importantly, can be reversed/halted when treating BP, especially with ACEi/ARB drugs and improved glycaemic control (Araki, et al., 2005; Hovind, et al., 2004; Perkins, et al., 2003).

People with hypertension

As discussed above, there is a case for screening for CKD in patients with hypertension. The UK CKD guidelines as well as the American KDOQI guidelines include hypertension as an indication for screening.

The British Hypertension Society guidelines recommend checking for proteinuria and eGFR at diagnosis followed by annual screening for proteinuria (Williams, et al., 2004).

Family history of CKD

There is an argument for including relatives of CKD patients in screening programmes. One study showed a high prevalence of CKD amongst relatives of patients with ESRD with 13.9% having a creatinine clearance of <60mL/min and 9.9% have +1 proteinuria or higher on dipstick (Jurkovitz, et al., 2008). Such rates are 2- to 3-fold higher than the general population. Another study looking at MA in relatives of CKD patients found that having a first-degree relative with CKD is associated with a seven times increase in the risk of MA (Bello, et al., 2008). Therefore, it would be advisable to screen relatives of patients with glomerulonephritis, diabetes, and hypertension for proteinuria.

Those suffering from obesity

Obesity is rapidly becoming the major global health care threat. Overweight and obesity affect more than 1.2 billion individual globally. There is also growing evidence associating obesity with the predisposition to and the progression of CKD. Obesity is also associated with MA as well as proteinuria. Therefore, screening for proteinuria in this group may prove to be cost-effective in preventing the progression to overt CKD.

Patients with CVD

CVD and CKD share a number of risk factors, including hypertension, hyperlipidaemia, and smoking. Therefore, the presence of atherosclerotic CVD is likely to be associated with atherosclerotic renovascular disease. In addition, heart failure is associated with reduced renal perfusion, and hence reduced GFR, and sometimes with proteinuria. It is not known whether screening for CKD in this group alters outcomes, but checking GFR is recommended as part of various aspects of management of CVD such as initiating and monitoring treatment with ACEi/ARB drugs.

The elderly

The prevalence of reduced GFR increases with age. Therefore, the number needed to screen to detect a case of CKD diminishes with age. Most of these data are based on the KDOQI classification whereby GFR $<60\text{mL/min}/1.73\text{m}^2$ is considered CKD stage 3. As alluded above, this cut-off is arbitrary and may not necessarily designate a 'disease' state or require any intervention. In fact there is evidence that elderly patients with CKD do not progress as fast as younger patients with CKD (Evans, et al., 2005). The UK CKD guidelines do not recommend routine screening in elderly patients, whereas the KDOQI guidelines recommend screening in people above the age of 60 years. If screening in the elderly is implemented, caution should be exerted, as mentioned above, to the potential misinterpretation of MA or reduced GFR in the elderly.

Race

There are clear ethnic differences in the incidence of ESRD. For example, data from the USRDS show that the incidence of ESRD in 2005 in white Americans was 286.4 per million population (pmp) compared to 769.6pmp in African Americans. Similar discrepancies are found in the UK between White and Asian populations.

The reasons for such a difference are beyond the scope of this article. However, despite this compelling evidence, current US and UK screening guidelines do not suggest screening in these ethnic groups.

Current screening guidelines

Most screening guidelines are consensus-based. There is not much in the way of hard evidence as most feasibility studies are based on hypothetical models.

International Society of Nephrology (ISN)

In 2004, following a wave of epidemiological studies screening for CKD using the KDOQI classification and for MA, the ISN called for mass population screening for albuminuria. This approach is also advocated by some groups, including de Jong and colleagues. They suggest screening for MA which would identify ~7% of the population as high risk of CKD and CVD and investigate those with high UAE with GFR estimation (de Jong, et al., 2008). However, as discussed above, MA is not specific for CKD and is variable, thus requiring repeated testing. Furthermore, only a small proportion of patients with advanced CKD have MA.

Current guidelines from different parts of the world do not support a mass population screening strategy, but recommend targeted screening, usually with eGFR. Examples of such guidelines are summarized below. They are mainly consensus-based and imply using eGFR as the screening method as they already target high-risk groups. They also lack details as to how often the screening should be repeated and whether the opportunist identification of 'at-risk groups' should be followed by entering those identified into a registry for subsequent screening. The cost-effectiveness of those strategies remains speculative because they lack detailed algorithms and/or mechanisms of implementation.

KDOQI

The American KDOQI guidelines (KDOQI, 2002) stipulate that all individuals should be assessed, as part of routine health encounters, to determine whether they are at increased risk of developing CKD, based on clinical and sociodemographic factors. Those include patients with diabetes mellitus, hypertension, autoimmune diseases, systemic infections, urinary tract infections, urological problems, and those treated with nephrotoxic drugs. The guidelines suggest screening using eGFR.

The UK CKD guidelines (NICE: National Institute for Health and Clinical Excellence guidelines)

Those recommend annual measurement of serum creatinine and estimating GFR in the following conditions: high risk of obstructive uropathy (e.g. neurogenic bladder), recurrent nephrolithiasis, hypertension, diabetes mellitus, heart failure, atherosclerotic vascular disease, and treatment with nephrotoxic medications such as ACEi, NSAIDs, and lithium, multisystem diseases, and first-degree relatives of CKD stage 5.

However, the UK CKD guidelines do not include screening the elderly (National Institute for Health and Clinical Excellence, 2008).

The Canadian Society of Nephrology

The Canadian Society of Nephrology also does not endorse mass population screening, but recommends case finding in those at risk, namely patients with diabetes, hypertension, heart failure, atherosclerotic vascular disease, unexplained anaemia, and 'First Nation people'. They recommend that those groups should have an eGFR and a PCR or an ACR (CSN, 2006).

Australian CARI (Caring for Australians with Renal Impairment) guidelines

Those guidelines suggest screening individuals with hypertension, vascular disease, or a family history of kidney disease using PCR as an initial screening test. They further suggest screening diabetics, Aborigines, and Torres Strait Islanders, more specifically using ACR (CARI, 2004).

Other strategies

Comparing guidelines

Table 4.6 gives a comparison of the screening programmes discussed above. To our knowledge, there are no mass population screening programmes in any country. The possible exception is Japan where all school children and all employees over the age of 40 are screened with urine dipstick. The health benefits of such strategy is uncertain (Iseki, 2006). Figure 4.1 gives a suggested practical scheme for screening for CKD.

One group from Norway, Hallan *et al.*, compared the sensitivity of the UK CKD guidelines and the KDOQI guidelines in detecting CKD if applied to the HUNT study population (Hallan, et al., 2006). They found that screening those with hypertension, diabetes, or age more that 55 would detect 93.2% of the population with eGFR <60, with the number needed to screen of 8.7 compared to 20.6 if mass population screening is applied. Those figures are similar if the KDOQI guidelines are applied. When the UK CKD guidelines are applied, only 60.9% of those with eGFR <60mL/min/1.73m^2 are identified. Obviously, the main difference that would account for the difference in sensitivity between the two sets of guidelines is incorporating age. Interestingly, Hallan *et al.*, with eight years follow-up data on their cohort, report that the risk of progression to ESRD from a baseline eGFR 45–59mL/min/1.73m^2 in non-diabetics, non-hypertensives, females, and over the age of 70 is particularly low. Therefore, one could argue, as we did above, that this group should not be labelled as having CKD.

Table 4.6 Comparison of different screening guidelines

Group	ISN	KDOQI	UK NICE	Canadian Society of Nephrology	CARI
Mass population	✓	✗	✗	✗	✗
Elderly	NA	✓ (over age of 60)	✗	✗	✗
Diabetes patients	NA	✓	✓	✓	✓*
Patients with hypertension	NA	✓	✓	✓	✓§
Patients with atherosclerotic vascular disease	NA	✗	✓	✓	✓§
Heart failure	NA	✗	✓	✓	✗
Urological conditions, e.g. obstruction, recurrent UTIs	NA	✓	✓	✗	✗
Autoimmune disease	NA	✓	✓	✓	✗
Nephrotoxic drugs	NA	✓	✓	✓	✗
Ethnic minorities	NA	✗	✗	✓	✓* (Aborigines and Torres Strait Islanders)
Relatives of CKD patients	NA	✗	✓	✗	✗
Test	Albuminuria	eGFR	eGFR	eGFR + ACR or PCR	PCR ACR
Frequency	NS	NS	Annual	NS	NS

✓=yes; ✗=no; NS=not specified; NA=not available; * ACR; §PCR

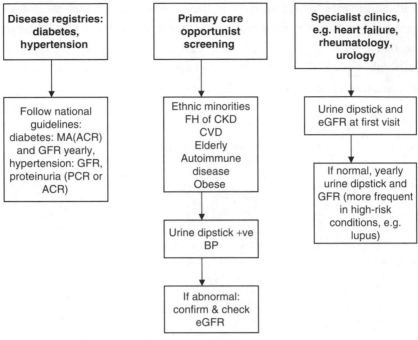

Fig. 4.1 Practical CKD screening recommendations

Conclusion

CKD is increasingly recognized in communities due to the systematic conversion of serum creatinine to estimated GFR. The majority of those found to have decreased eGFR are over the age of 60. Caution should be applied in the interpretation of eGFR values in the elderly as a significant percentage may have an age-related decline in kidney function without the implications normally associated with progressive CKD. In the younger population, it is advisable to attempt detecting those with proteinuria and/or declining GFR (<60mL/min/1.73m^2) as those are at higher risk of progression to ESRD and are also at a higher CVD morbidity and mortality risk. The majority will have associated diabetes and/or hypertension. Attention should focus on these individuals as interventions based on the control of glycaemia, hypertension as well as the inhibition of the RAAS have proven to be protective. Detection of CKD in these individuals would serve the dual purpose of slowing the progression of CKD and reducing cardiovascular complications. The latter would also be enhanced by the control of dyslipidaemia and cessation of smoking. Therefore, we advocate a focused and targeted approach to CKD screening and detection. Such an approach should be cost-effective and affordable to high as well as low economies.

References

Araki, S., Haneda, M., Sugimoto, T., Isono, M., Isshiki, K., Kashiwagi, A., Koya, D., 2005. Factors associated with frequent remission of microalbuminuria in patients with type 2 diabetes. *Diabetes*, 54(10), pp.2983–7.

Arnlov, J., Evans, J.C., Meigs, J.B., Wang, T.J., Fox, C.S., Levy, D., Benjamin, E.J., D'Agostino, R.B., Vasan, R.S., 2005. Low-grade albuminuria and incidence of cardiovascular disease events in nonhypertensive and nondiabetic individuals: the Framingham Heart Study. *Circulation*, 112(7), pp.969–75.

Atkins, R.C., Briganti, E.M., Lewis, J.B., Hunsicker, L.G., Braden, G., Champion de Crespigny, P.J., DeFerrari, G., Drury, P., Locatelli, F., Wiegmann, T.B., Lewis, E.J., 2005. Proteinuria reduction and progression to renal failure in patients with type 2 diabetes mellitus and overt nephropathy. *American Journal of Kidney Diseases*, 45(2), pp.281–7.

Bello, A., Peters, J., Wight, J., De Zeeuw, D., El Nahas, M.; European Kidney Institute, 2008. A population-based screening for microalbuminuria among relatives of CKD patients: The kidney evaluation and awareness program in Sheffield (KEAPS). *American Journal of Kidney Diseases*, 52(3), pp.434–43.

Borch–Johnsen, K., Feldt–Rasmussen, B., Strandgaard, S., Schroll, M., Jensen, J.S., 1999. Urinary albumin excretion. An independent predictor of ischemic heart disease. *Arteriosclerosis, thrombosis, and vascular biology*, 19(8), pp.1992–7.

Boulware, L.E., Jaar, B.G., Tarver–Carr, M.E., Brancati, F.L., Powe, N.R., 2003. Screening for proteinuria in US adults: a cost-effectiveness analysis. *Journal of the American Medical Association*, 290(23), pp.3101–14.

Caring for Australians with Renal Impairment, 2004. *Testing for proteinuria*. [Online] Available at: http://www.cari.org.au Accessed June 2008.

Chen, J., Wildman, R.P., Gu, D., Kusek, J.W., Spruill, M., Reynolds, K., Liu, D., Hamm, L.L., Whelton, P.K., He, J., 2005. Prevalence of decreased kidney function in Chinese adults aged 35 to 74 years. *Kidney International*, 68(6), pp.2837–45.

Cockcroft, D.W., Gault, M.H., 1976. Prediction of creatinine clearance from serum creatinine. *Nephron*, 16(1), pp.31–41.

Coresh, J., Selvin, E., Stevens, L.A., Manzi, J., Kusek, J.W., Eggers, P., Van Lente, F., Levey, A.S., 2007. Prevalence of Chronic Kidney Disease in the United States. *Journal of the American Medical Association*, 298(17), pp.2038–47.

Craig, J.C., Barratt, A., Cumming, R., Irwig, L., Salkeld, G., 2002. Feasibility study of the early detection and treatment of renal disease by mass screening. *Internal Medicine Journal*, 32(1–2), pp.6–14.

Datta, M., Mani, M.K., 2006. Community-based approach to prevention of chronic kidney disease. In: El Nahas, A.M., ed. *Kidney diseases in the developing world and ethnic minorities*. New York: Taylor and Francis, pp.393–411.

de Jong, P.E., van der Velde, M., Gansevoort, R.T., Zoccali, C., 2008. Screening for chronic kidney disease: where does Europe go? *Clinical Journal of the American Society of Nephrology*, 3(2), pp.616–23.

Dinneen, S.F., Gerstein, H.C., 1997. The association of microalbuminuria and mortality in non-insulin-dependent diabetes mellitus. A systematic overview of the literature. *Archives of internal medicine*, 157(13), pp.1413–8.

Dyer, A.R., Greenland, P., Elliott, P., Daviglus, M.L., Claeys, G., Kesteloot, H., Ueshima, H., Stamler, J; INTERMAP Research Group, 2004. Evaluation of measures of urinary albumin excretion in epidemiologic studies. *American Journal of Epidemiology*, 160(11), pp.1122–31.

Evans, M., Fryzek, J.P., Elinder, C.G., Cohen, S.S., McLaughlin, J.K., Nyren, O., Fored, C.M., 2005. The natural history of chronic renal failure: results from an unselected, population-based, inception cohort in Sweden. *American Journal of Kidney Diseases*, 46(5), pp.863–70.

Foley, R.N., Wang, C., Ishani, A., Ibrahim, H.N., Collins, A.J., 2008. Creatinine-based glomerular filtration rates and microalbuminuria for detecting metabolic abnormalities in US adults: the National Health and Nutrition Examination Survey 2003–2004. *American Journal of Nephrology*, 28(3), pp.431–7.

Froissart, M., Rossert, J., Jacquot, C., Paillard, M., Houillier, P., 2005. Predictive performance of the modification of diet in renal disease and Cockcroft–Gault equations for estimating renal function. Journal of the American Society of *Nephrology*, 16(3), pp.763–73.

Garg, A.X., Kiberd, B.A., Clark, W.F., Haynes, R.B., Clase, C.M., 2002. Albuminuria and renal insufficiency prevalence guides population screening: results from the NHANES III. *Kidney International*, 61(6), pp.2165–75.

Go, A.S., Chertow, G.M., Fan, D., McCulloch, C.E., Hsu, C.Y., 2004. Chronic kidney disease and the risks of death, cardiovascular events, and hospitalization. *New England Journal of Medicine*, 351(13), pp.1296–1305.

Hallan, S.I., Dahl, K., Oien, C.M., Grootendorst, D.C., Aasberg, A, Holmen, J., Dekker, F.W., 2006. Screening strategies for chronic kidney disease in the general population: follow-up of cross sectional health survey. *British Medical Journal*, 333(7577), p.1047.

Henry, R.M., Kostense, P.J., Bos, G., Dekker, J.M., Nijpels, G., Heine, R.J., Bouter, L.M., Stehouwer, C.D., 2002. Mild renal insufficiency is associated with increased cardiovascular mortality: the Hoorn Study. *Kidney International*, 62(4), pp.1402–7.

Hillege, H.L., Fidler, V., Diercks, G.F., van Gilst, W.H., de Zeeuw, D., van Veldhuisen, D.J., Gans, R.O., Janssen, W.M., Grobbee, D.E., de Jong, P.E.;

Prevention of Renal and Vascular End Stage Disease (PREVEND) Study Group, 2002. Urinary albumin excretion predicts cardiovascular and non-cardiovascular mortality in general population. *Circulation*, 106(14), pp.1777–82.

Hovind, P., Tarnow, L., Rossing, P., Jensen, B.R., Graae, M., Torp, I., Binder, C., Parvinig, H.H., 2004. Predictors for the development of microalbuminuria and macroalbuminuria in patients with type 1 diabetes: inception cohort study. *British Medical Journal*, 328(7448), p.1105.

Iseki, K., 2006. Screening for renal disease–what can be learned from the Okinawa experience. *Nephrology Dialysis Transplantation*, 21(4), pp.839–43.

Iseki, K., Iscki, C., Ikemiya, Y., Fukiyama, K., 1996. Risk of developing end-stage renal disease in a cohort of mass screening. *Kidney International*, 49(3), pp.800–5.

Jafar, T.H., Stark, P.C., Schmid, C.H., Landa, M., Maschio, G., Marcantoni, C., de Jong, P.E., de Zeeuw, D., Shahinfar, S., Ruggenenti, P., Remuzzi, G., Levey, A.S., AIPRD Study Group. Angiotensin-Converting Enzyme Inhibition, and Progression of Renal Disease, 2001. Proteinuria as a modifiable risk factor for the progression of non-diabetic renal disease. *Kidney International*, 60(3), pp.1131–40.

Jurkovitz, C.T., Qiu, Y., Wang, C., Gilbertson, D.T., Brown, W.W., 2008. The Kidney Early Evaluation Program (KEEP): program design and demographic characteristics of the population. *American Journal of Kidney Diseases*, 51(4 Suppl 2), S3–12.

KDOQI, 2002. Clinical practice guidelines for chronic kidney disease: evaluation, classification, and stratification. *American Journal of Kidney Diseases*, 39(2 Suppl 1), S1–266.

Klahr, S., Levey, A.S., Beck, G.J., Caggiula, A.W., Hunsicker, L., Kusek, J.W., Striker, G., 1994. The effects of dietary protein restriction and blood-pressure control on the progression of chronic renal disease. Modification of Diet in Renal Disease Study Group. *New England Journal of Medicine*, 330(13), pp.877–84.

Konta, T., Hao, Z., Abiko, H., Ishikawa, M., Takahashi, T., Ikeda, A., Ichikawa, K., Takasaki, S., Kubota, I., 2006. Prevalence and risk factor analysis of microalbuminuria in Japanese general population: the Takahata study. *Kidney International*, 70(4), pp.751–6.

Lameire, N., Jager, K., Van Biesen, W., de Bacquer, D., Vanholder, R., 2005. Chronic kidney disease: a European perspective. *Kidney International Suppl*, (99), S30–8.

Lea, J., Greene, T., Hebert, L., Lipkowitz, M., Massry, S., Middleton, J., Rostand, S.G., Miller, E., Smith, W., Bakris, G.L., 2005. The relationship between magnitude of proteinuria reduction and risk of end-stage renal disease: results of the African American study of kidney disease and hypertension. *Archives of Internal Medicine*, 165(8), pp.947–53.

Levey, A.S., Bosch, J.P., Lewis, J.B., Greene, T., Rogers, N., Roth, D., 1999. A more accurate method to estimate glomerular filtration rate from serum creatinine: a new prediction equation. Modification of Diet in Renal Disease Study Group. *Annals of Internal Medicine*, 130(6), pp.461–70.

Locatelli, F., Marcelli, D., Comelli, M., Alberti, D., Graziani, G., Buccianti, G., Redaelli, B., Giangrande, A., 1996. Proteinuria and blood pressure as causal components of progression to end-stage renal failure. Northern Italian Cooperative Study Group. *Nephrology Dialysis Transplantation*, 11(3), pp.461–7.

Marshall, S.M., 1991. Screening for microalbuminuria: which measurement? *Diabetic Medicine*, 8(8), pp.706–11.

Mogensen, C.E., 1984. Microalbuminuria predicts clinical proteinuria and early mortality in maturity-onset diabetes. *New England Journal of Medicine*, 310(6), pp.356–60.

National Institute for Health and Clinical Excellence, 2008. Early identification and management of chronic kidney disease in adults in primary and secondary care. (http://guidance.nice.org.uk/CG73) Accessed March 2009.

Perkins, B.A., Ficociello, L.H., Silva, K.H., Finkelstein, D.M., Warram, J.H., Krolewski, A.S., 2003. Regression of microalbuminuria in type 1 diabetes. *New England Journal of Medicine*, 348(23), pp.2285–93.

Peterson, J., Adler, S., Burkart, J., Greene, T., Herbert, L.A., Hunsicker, L.G., King, A.J., Klahr, S., Massry, S.G., Seifter, J.L., 1995. Blood pressure control, proteinuria, and the progression of renal disease: The Modification of Diet in Renal Disease Study. *Annals in Internal Medicine*, 123(10), pp.754–62.

Romundstad, S., Holmen, J., Kvenild, K., Hallan, H., Ellekjaer, H., 2003. Microalbuminuria and all-cause mortality in 2,089 apparently healthy individuals: a 4.4-year follow-up study. The Nord-Trondelag Health Study (HUNT), Norway. *American Journal of Kidney Diseases*, 42(3), pp.466–73.

Siedner, M.J., Gelber, A.C., Rovin, B.H., McKinley, A.M., Christopher–Stine, L., Astor, B., Petri, M., Fine, D.M., 2008. Diagnostic accuracy study of urine dipstick in relation to 24-hour measurement as a screening tool for proteinuria in lupus nephritis. *Journal of Rheumatology*, 35(1), pp.84–90.

Stack, A.G., 2003. Impact of timing of nephrology referral and pre-ESRD care on mortality risk among new ESRD patients in the United States. *American Journal of Kidney Diseases*, 41(2), pp.310–8.

Strippoli, G.F., Navaneethan, S.D., Johnson, D.W., Perkovic, V., Pellegrini, F., Nicolucci, A., Craig, J.C., 2008. Effects of statins in patients with chronic kidney disease: meta-analysis and meta-regression of randomised controlled trials. *British Medical Journal*, 336(7645), pp.645–51.

The Canadian Society of Nephrology, 2006. *Detection, monitoring and referral of CKD*. [Online] Available at: http://csnscn.ca/english/professional%20practice/guidelines/implementationcommittee/ Accessed June 2008.

United States Renal Data System, 2003. *Annual report 2003*. [Online]

Available at: http://www.usrds.org/adr_2003.htm Accessed June 2008.

Verhave, J.C., Gansevoort, R.T., Hillege, H.L., Bakker, S.J., De Zeeuw, D., de Jong, P.E., 2004. An elevated urinary albumin excretion predicts de novo development of renal function impairment in the general population. *Kidney International Suppl*, (92), S18–21.

Viberti, G.C., Hill, R.D., Jarrett, R.J., Argyropoulos, A., Mahmud, U., Keen, H., 1982. Microalbuminuria as a predictor of clinical nephropathy in insulin-dependent diabetes mellitus. *Lancet*, 1(8287), pp.1430–2.

Williams, B., Poulter, N.R., Brown, M.J., Davis, M., McInnes, G.T., Potter, J.F., Sever, P.S., Thom, S.M.; BHS guidelines working party, for the British Hypertension Society, 2004. British Hypertension Society guidelines for hypertension management 2004 (BHS-IV): summary. *British Medical Journal*, 328(7440), pp.634–40.

Wilson, J.M., Jungner, Y.G., 1968. [Principles and practice of mass screening for disease]. *Boletin de la Oficina Sanitaria Panamericana*, 65(4): pp.281–393.

Yudkin, J.S., Forrest, R.D., Jackson, C.A., 1988. Microalbuminuria as predictor of vascular disease in non-diabetic subjects. Islington Diabetes Survey. *Lancet*, 2(8610), pp.530–3.

Yuyun, M.F., Khaw, K.T., Luben, R., Welch, A., Bingham, S., Day, N.E., Wareham, N.J., 2004. A prospective study of microalbuminuria and incident coronary heart disease and its prognostic significance in a British population: the EPIC-Norfolk study. *American Journal of Epidemiology*, 159(3), pp.284–93.

Chapter 5

Chronic kidney disease and cardiovascular disease

Daniel E. Weiner and Mark J. Sarnak

Introduction

Chronic kidney disease (CKD) is a potentially progressive condition marked by either reduced kidney function or the presence of kidney damage. Kidney function is quantified by the glomerular filtration rate (GFR), often estimated with equations that use serum creatinine and demographic characteristics. The early stages of CKD (stages 1 and 2) are defined by kidney damage (most often manifest with microalbuminuria) in the presence of intact GFR ($>60mL/min/1.73m^2$), while later stages (stages 3 and 4) are associated with decreased GFR. In an individual with progressive kidney disease, kidney failure (CKD stage 5) ensues and renal replacement therapy (RRT) is required. However, most people with CKD never reach kidney failure; rather, they die prematurely of cardiovascular disease (CVD). Therefore, major therapeutic goals in individuals with CKD, aside from preventing the progression to kidney failure, include the recognition of increased cardiovascular risk and treatment of CVD risk factors and manifestations. In this section, we will discuss CKD as a risk state for CVD, describe factors that are associated with higher cardio-vascular risk in individuals with CKD, review the aetiology, diagnosis. and treatment of CVD in patients with CKD, and discuss CVD as a risk factor for CKD. Key factors relevant to the primary and secondary management of CVD in patients with advanced CKD are presented in Table 5.1.

Kidney disease: cardiovascular risk factor?

CVD risk factors are defined as characteristics, both modifiable and non-modifiable, that increase the risk of developing CVD; these include both traditional and non-traditional risk factors.

Table 5.1 Key points for cardiovascular care in patients with CKD

CVD is very common in patients with CKD.

CKD may be considered a CVD risk equivalent.

There is a wide spectrum of CVD, all of which is highly prevalent in patients with CKD, including atherosclerosis, arteriosclerosis, LVH and heart failure, valvular disease, and arrhythmias.

Increased risk of CVD events is seen in patients with an eGFR <60 and/or in the presence of even small amount of protein in the urine.

A 20-year old dialysis patient has an equivalent cardiovascular risk to an 80-year old not on dialysis.

CVD is understudied in patients with CKD.

Patients with reduced kidney function are excluded from many clinical trials.

Most recommendations for management are based on limited data extrapolated from the non-CKD population.

CVD is under-treated in patients with CKD.

CKD patients are less likely to receive appropriate medications following a myocardial infarction and are less likely to receive revascularization therapies.

CVD is treatable in patients with CKD.

Prevention may be accomplished through BP, diabetes, and lipid management as well as possible benefits with the management of other risk factors.

Treatment with the above as well as anti-platelet agents, coronary revascularization, and other therapeutics are similar to that in non-CKD.

Very few medications are contraindicated in CKD, but many require dosing adjustments.

There is minimal data on how to best treat dialysis patients.

In dialysis patients, several medications should be avoided (e.g. atenolol, eptifibatide) or used with caution and careful attention to dose adjustment (e.g. digoxin, enoxaparin, tirofiban).

Table 5.2 Traditional and non-traditional CVD risk factors. Adapted with permission from Sarnak, et al., 2003.

Traditional risk factors	Non-traditional risk factors
Older age	Albuminuria
Male sex	Lipoprotein a and Apo a isoforms
Hypertension	Lipoprotein remnants
Elevated LDL cholesterol	Anaemia
Low HDL cholesterol	Abnormal mineral metabolism
Diabetes mellitus	Volume overload
Smoking	Electrolyte imbalances
Physical inactivity	Oxidative stress/inflammation
Menopause	Malnutrition
Family history of CVD	Thrombogenic factors
LVH	Sleep disturbances
Obesity	Altered nitric oxide/endothelin balance

Traditional CVD risk factors

These were identified in the Framingham Heart Study and form the basis of prediction equations to aid physicians in identifying individuals at higher risk of CVD. These include older age, male sex, hypertension, diabetes, smoking, and family history of coronary disease, and are summarized in Table 5.2 (Sarnak, et al., 2003).

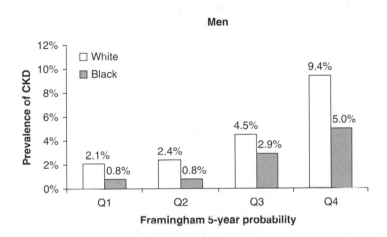

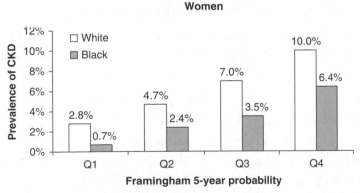

Fig. 5.1 The prevalence of CKD based on the quartile of the Framingham risk score for developing coronary heart disease within five years, stratified by race in men and women. The p value for trend within each sex-specific race group is <0.001.

Reprinted with permission from Weiner, et al., 2007.

- Traditional CVD risk factors are highly prevalent in individuals with CKD (Figure 5.1).

- Equations derived from the general population using traditional risk factors do not accurately predict CVD outcomes in later stages (3–4) of CKD and dialysis.

Non-traditional CVD risk factors

These were not described in the original Framingham studies. They are defined as risk factors that increase in prevalence as the kidney function declines and are associated with CVD, and they are summarized in Table 5.2.

- Several risk factors, including anaemia and abnormalities in mineral metabolism, are particular to individuals with CKD.

- Other risk factors, including inflammation and oxidative stress, are considered important in all populations.

The role of CKD as an independent risk state for CVD

This has been investigated in several studies, with the majority focusing on either reduced GFR (<60mL/min/1.73m^2) or the presence of albuminuria after accounting for traditional CVD risk factors.

Kidney function (CKD stages 3–4) and CVD risk

- Individuals with an estimated GFR (eGFR) <60mL/min/1.73m^2 have many more CVD events and higher mortality rates than those without a reduced kidney function (Figure 5.2).

- Most, but not all cohort studies, note a relatively robust association between reduced eGFR and subsequent CVD, even after adjusting for traditional CVD risk factors, particularly in populations that include African Americans and in populations evaluating recurrent cardiovascular events (Go, et al., 2004; Weiner, et al., 2006).

- A meta-analysis of 39 community-based studies that followed a total of 1,371,990 participants demonstrated an increased risk of all-cause mortality associated with an eGFR <60mL/min/1.73m^2 in 71% of these cohorts (Tonelli, et al., 2006).

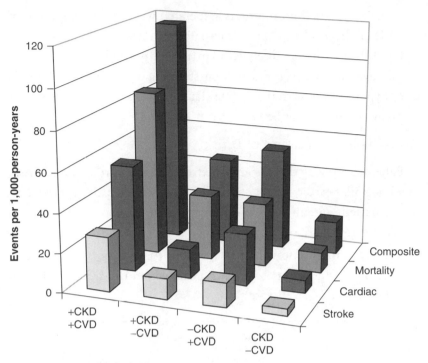

Fig. 5.2 Event rates for individuals with and without CKD and CVD. Cardiac events include myocardial infarction and fatal coronary disease. Stroke includes both fatal and non-fatal stroke events. Mortality includes all causes of death and the composite outcome includes any cardiac, stroke, or mortality event.

Reprinted with the permission of the National Kidney Foundation from Weiner, et al., 2006.

Albuminuria and CVD risk

- Albuminuria refers to albumin leakage into the urine and to account for urine being concentrated or dilute, it is commonly reported as the ratio of urine albumin to urine creatinine.
  - Microalbuminuria, defined by a urine albumin-to-creatinine ratio (ACR) of 30–300mg/g, often marks early kidney damage due to diabetes, hypertension, or other conditions.
  - Macroalbuminuria, defined by an ACR exceeding 300mg/g, is often seen in more advanced diabetic or hypertensive kidney disease, or in primary or secondary glomerular diseases.
- Multiple studies have demonstrated that the presence of even very small amounts of albumin in the urine, below the threshold defined

as being microalbuminuria, is associated with the development of CVD (Hillege, et al., 2002). Microalbuminuria is unlikely to cause CVD, but rather is likely to identify individuals with systemic microvascular damage due to long-standing or more severe diabetes or hypertension, with the glomerular capillaries merely being one of many target vascular beds.

Kidney failure/ESRD and CVD risk

• Patients receiving dialysis are at extremely high cardiovascular risk, with similar cardiovascular mortality rates seen in a 20-year old dialysis patient and an 80-year old member of the general population (Figure 5.3) (Sarnak & Levey, 2000).

  • CVD is highly prevalent in incident dialysis patients (at least 22.5% of individuals initiating dialysis in the US in 2006 had known coronary disease).

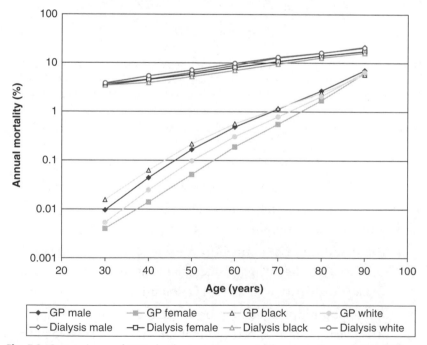

Fig. 5.3 Comparisons of CVD death at a given age in the general population (GP) and the ESRD population.

Reprinted from *American Journal of Kidney Diseases*, 32, Foley, R.N., Parfrey, P.S., Sarnak, M.J., The clinical epidemiology of cardiovascular disease in chronic renal disease, S112–S119, 1998 (Suppl 3), with permission from Elsevier.

- There is a high case fatality rate for incident CVD in dialysis patients as compared to the general population (Herzog, et al., 1998).
- Subclinical coronary disease also may be highly prevalent (Ohtake, et al., 2005).

Identifying those individuals with CKD who are at highest risk of ischaemic heart disease: markers and equations

The Framingham prediction equations utilize traditional risk factors, including age, sex, blood pressure (BP), diabetes, smoking, and lipid levels to estimate cardiac risk in a general US population. Use of these well-accepted prediction equations may be problematic in patients with CKD as altered risk factor relationships are prevalent in CKD such that typical risk factors, even those where good causal models exist for causing CVD, may appear protective. This has been dubbed 'reverse epidemiology' by some researchers.

In dialysis, risk factors that are dependent on intact nutrition such as higher cholesterol and risk factors dependent on cardiac and cardiovascular health such as higher systolic and diastolic BP appear protective.

- For example, there is little increase in mortality risk at even the highest systolic BP while lower systolic BP (<120mmHg) are associated with the highest risk of mortality (Kalantar–Zadeh, et al., 2003).
- Accordingly, Framingham equations fail altogether in dialysis, although older individuals and those with diabetes do have higher cardiovascular event rates.
- In CKD, most traditional risk factors that predict coronary heart disease in the general population remain important risk factors.
  - The relative importance of each risk factor may be different; for example, diabetes in individuals with an eGFR <60mL/min/1.73m^2 is a more powerful marker of cardiac risk than it is in the general population, perhaps reflecting the fact that diabetes severe enough to cause kidney damage is also capable of causing systemic vascular disease.

Causes, diagnosis, and treatment of CVD in CKD

CVD in individuals with CKD, similar to the general population, can be broadly classified into arterial disease, cardiomyopathy, other structural heart diseases, including valvular and pericardial disease, and arrhythmias. Each of these categories has factors that are distinct to CKD. While this chapter focuses on cardiac disease, the pathophysiology is similar across the entire vasculature.

Ischaemic heart disease

Aetiology of ischaemic heart disease

Arterial disease in individuals with CKD can be broadly classified as relating to **atherosclerosis**, a focal process of plaque formation resulting in luminal narrowing, and **arteriosclerosis**, a diffuse process of arterial stiffening resulting in increased systolic BP and pulse pressure as well as compensatory left ventricular hypertrophy in the setting of increased afterload (Table 5.3). In most cases, it is the interplay between atherosclerosis and arteriosclerosis that yields clinically apparent ischaemic CVD (London, et al., 2002).

Atherosclerosis and arteriosclerosis   Atherosclerosis in CKD has been dubbed 'accelerated' in efforts to explain the high prevalence.

- It represents the manifestation of increasingly severe risk factors, most notably hypertension, in the setting of fluid retention and a highly atherogenic lipid profile. For example, while the level of low density lipoprotein (LDL) cholesterol may appear normal in CKD, increased oxidized LDL cholesterol, triglycerides and lipoprotein a, and lower HDL cholesterol are common findings, both in the presence and absence of nephrotic range proteinuria.

Arteriosclerosis is synonymous with arterial stiffness and represents a state of reduced arterial compliance.

- Commonly occurs in aging, but is far more profound in CKD, potentially related to the high prevalence of hypertension as well as disorders of mineral metabolism promoting arterial calcification.
  - Onset in the early stages of CKD.
  - Manifests with increased pulse pressure.

Table 5.3 Causes, risk factors, and manifestations of arterial disease in CKD

Classification	Notable risk factors	Indicators/ diagnostic test	Clinical sequelae
Atherosclerosis Luminal narrowing of arteries due to plaques In advanced CKD, plaques often highly calcified	Traditional risk factors (e.g. dyslipidaemia, diabetes, hypertension, smoking) Non-traditional risk factors (e.g. endothelial dysfunction, inflammation)	Inducible ischaemia on nuclear imaging or stress echocardiogram Cardiac catheterization Carotid intima-media thickness Coronary ultrasound Coronary computed tomography	Myocardial infarction Angina Sudden cardiac death Heart failure Stroke Peripheral vascular disease
Arteriosclerosis Diffuse dilatation and wall hypertrophy of larger arteries Loss of arterial elasticity and compliance	Hypertension Volume overload Hyperparathyroidism Hyperphosphataemia	Vascular calcification Increased pulse pressure Aortic pulse wave velocity Coronary computed tomography	Higher systolic BP Higher pulse pressure Myocardial infarction Angina Sudden cardiac death Heart failure LVH

- May be more precisely assessed with measures of aortic pulse wave velocity (PWV) and augmentation index (AI), both of which are associated with increased mortality in dialysis patients.
- Promoted by the dialysis milieu as demonstrated by the presence of markedly increased PWV and AI in children receiving dialysis.

Potential non-traditional mediators of atherosclerosis and arteriosclerosis in CKD   The mineral and bone disorder of CKD may result in CKD through arteriosclerosis (Brosius, et al., 2006).

- Vascular calcification occurs in both the arterial tunica media (arteriosclerosis) as well as the tunica intima (atherosclerosis) in CKD.
  - More common in individuals with reduced kidney function (CKD stage 3 or higher) than in the general population, likely reflecting a complex interrelationship among hyperphosphataemia, secondary

hyperparathyroidism, vitamin D deficiency, and other more novel markers of mineral metabolism, including increased fibroblast growth factor (FGF)-23 and decreased fetuin A (El-Abbadi & Giachelli, 2007).

- Vascular calcification, in the forms of coronary artery calcification and both peripheral artery intimal and medial calcification, is independently associated with mortality in dialysis patients.

- Whether vascular calcification is causal or merely a marker of vascular burden is unknown, with this uncertainty bolstered by a lack of a consistent dose-effect response between GFR and coronary calcification, and the absence of a robust association between reduced kidney function and coronary calcification after adjusting for traditional cardiovascular risk factors and inflammation.

Inflammation represents an attractive, unifying hypothesis for the high prevalence of CVD seen in all stages of CKD (Himmelfarb, et al., 2002).

- The lesions of atherosclerosis in large part represent a sequence of inflammatory processes affecting the vasculature as elevated and modified LDL cholesterol, genetic factors, infectious microorganisms, free radicals caused by cigarette smoking, hypertension, diabetes mellitus and ischaemic injury, and combinations of these all predispose to progressive endothelial dysfunction.

- Individuals with CKD have multiple potential inflammatory stimuli, including ischaemia, infection, and the uraemic milieu.

- An imbalance in pro- and antioxidant agents exists in CKD, perhaps mediated by impaired pro-inflammatory cytokine clearance, and may contribute.

- In the general population, inflammation is a reasonably well-established risk marker for CVD, with leukocytosis and C-reactive protein (CRP) both independently associated with adverse cardiovascular outcomes.

- This also appears to be the case in individuals with a reduced kidney function.

◆ Notably, there is no significant difference in the magnitude of risks associated with inflammatory markers when comparing individuals with an eGFR below and above 60mL/min/1.73m^2, implying a lack of synergistic CVD risk enhancement between inflammation and CKD.

Anaemia is common in individuals with advanced CKD and kidney failure and may be associated with CVD.

◆ In an observational study, individuals with CDK stages 3–4 with both anaemia and left ventricular hypertrophy had a substantially increased risk of cardiac events and mortality.

◆ Similarly, the concurrent presence of anaemia and CKD stages 3–4 led to a significantly increased risk of cardiac and mortality events, particularly in individuals with diabetes.

◆ In individuals with systolic heart failure, anaemia is associated with a more rapid decline in GFR and in those with concurrent heart failure and CKD, anaemia is associated with an increased all-cause mortality.

Diagnosis of ischaemic heart disease

The diagnosis of ischaemic heart disease, particularly in the absence of acute electrocardiogram changes, is a challenge in the CKD population. There is no single test for identifying ischaemic heart disease in patients with CKD, and each test currently used to identify cardiac ischaemia has disadvantages specific to CKD that may affect sensitivity and specificity.

Functional assessments may provide the best assessment of cardiac ischaemia.

◆ Exercise or pharmacologic nuclear stress tests.

◆ Exercise or pharmacologic stress echocardiography may be particularly useful as echocardiography also provides information on valvular and other structural disease.

• Limited role for stress electrocardiography (ECG) in this population given the high prevalence of baseline ECG abnormalities and CVD.

- ◆ Coronary angiography should be used as indicated, despite individuals with CKD representing a higher risk population for complications of angiography, including bleeding and re-stenosis with or without stenting.
  - • Critically, the preservation of existing kidney function is an important consideration in all stages of kidney disease, including for those receiving dialysis, and with careful management and conservative use of iodinated contrast, many individuals with CKD stages 3 and 4 can avoid significant contrast nephropathy.

Laboratory evaluation of coronary syndromes in CKD patients also is challenging, as many of the markers used in the general population, including cardiac troponins I and T, N-terminal pro-B-type natriuretic peptide (NT-proBNP), creatine kinase (CK) and the MB subfraction of creatine kinase (CK-MB), and myoglobin may be chronically elevated. For example, 20% of asymptomatic haemodialysis patients have cardiac troponin T levels that would be consistent with an acute myocardial infarction in the general population (>0.1μg/L) (Apple, et al., 2002).

- ◆ In the setting of mild to moderate elevation of cardiac markers, the identification of an acute coronary syndrome in the absence of a suggestive ECG should utilize data on changes in the levels of these markers.
- ◆ Prognostic importance is attached to chronic elevation of cardiac markers.
  - • Chronic elevation of troponin T predicts mortality in both CKD stages 3–4 and dialysis patients, identifying patients with greater left ventricular dilatation as well as impaired left ventricular systolic and diastolic function.
  - • Elevations in NT-proBNP predict underlying ischaemic heart disease and hypertrophy, independent of the level of kidney function.

Prevention and treatment of ischaemic heart disease: Stages 3–4 CKD

In **CKD stages 3–4**, therapeutic data are lacking, predominantly reflecting the fact that many studies have excluded participants with an elevated serum creatinine. Therefore, we are mostly reliant on post hoc subgroup analyses derived from larger clinical trials that had serum creatinine cut-offs of 2 or 3mg/dL for inclusion. In general, most of these studies demonstrate benefits for CKD stages 3–4 patients that are similar to those appreciated in the general population, and treatment strategies for the primary prevention of cardiac disease in individuals with CKD mirror those seen in the general population (KDOQI, 2005; Tonelli, et al., 2004). Therapeutic targets for individuals with CKD not receiving kidney replacement therapies are summarized in Table 5.4.

Challenges specific to the Stage 3–4 CKD population

- More frequent hyperkalaemia impacting the use of ACE inhibitors (ACEis), angiotensin receptor blockers (ARBs), and spironolactone.
- Increased risk of rhabdomyolysis seen with statin and fibrate therapy.
  - Concurrent use of statins and fibrates should be avoided in advanced CKD.

Therapeutic targets in Stages 3–4 CKD BP should be <130/80mmHg.

- In the presence of macroalbuminuria, strong evidence exists supporting the use of an ACEi or ARB as a first-line agent to achieve BP control and these medications will typically be accompanied by a diuretic.
- In the absence of albuminuria in patients without diabetes, ACEis and ARBs may be preferable to other agents, but the evidence is scant. Accordingly, BP treatment choices in these individuals may favour beta-blockade in an individual requiring secondary prevention following a myocardial infarction.
- In many individuals with CKD stage 3 and nearly all individuals with stage 4, a thiazide diuretic will have minimal BP efficacy and a loop diuretic may be preferable.
- Patients with CKD often will require four or more drugs to achieve this BP goal.
- Dietary counselling, particularly sodium reduction, may have a substantial impact on BP control, given the net positive sodium balance often seen in later stages of CKD.

Table 5.4 Treatment goals for primary and secondary prevention of ischaemic CVD in CKD stages 3–4

Risk factor	Action plan
BP	Target <130/80mmHg based on JNC 7 guidelines
	ACEi or ARB if ACEi not tolerated are first-line agents in patients with albuminuria or diabetes
	Diuretics often required, and thiazides will have decreased efficacy in late stage CKD
	Four or more medications often needed to achieve target
	Possible benefit to targeting even lower BP in individuals with proteinuria
	Atenolol should be avoided in kidney failure
Dyslipidaemia	Target LDL cholesterol <100mg/dL
	Lifestyle changes should be attempted, but often are unsuccessful
	Statins are safe and effective for LDL reduction and are first-line for treating elevated LDL cholesterol
	Fibrates, specifically gemfibrozil, are first-line for patients with triglycerides >500mg/dL
	Concurrent use of statins and fibrates should be avoided in late stage CKD due to a high risk of rhabdomyolysis
Smoking	Smoking cessation methods as attempted in the general population
Diabetes	Glycosylated haemoglobin target of <7%
	Glipizide is the preferred sulfonylurea
	Insulin often required
	Metformin should be avoided
Anti-platelet therapy	Aspirin may be used for both primary and secondary prevention, with contraindications identical to those in the general population
Anaemia	Current KDOQI target haemoglobin level is 11–12g/dL
	US Food and Drug Administration suggest adjusting epoetin dosing to maintain haemoglobin level of 10–12g/dL
	No data demonstrating improved survival
Obesity	Obesity management as attempted in the general population
	Potential role for bariatric surgery

Dyslipidaemia treatment goals are similar to the general population with several guideline development groups classifying CKD as a cardiac risk equivalent (similar to diabetes). The best evidence to date is derived from a recent meta-analysis of 50 placebo-controlled trials analyzing the subgroup of patients in larger trials with GFR <60mL/min/1.73m^2.

This meta-analysis showed a significant reduction associated with statins in fatal and non-fatal cardiovascular events; however, statins had no significant effect on all-cause mortality (Strippoli, et al., 2008). Meta-regression analysis showed that treatment effects did not vary significantly with CKD stage. Treatment goals and regimens are described below:

- Therapeutic lifestyle changes (TLC) remain an essential modality in clinical management.
- Treatment goal of LDL cholesterol <100mg/dL is reasonable, based on data from the general population and is primarily accomplished with statins.
  - To date, there is inadequate data to support an LDL cholesterol goal of <70mg/dL in individuals with CKD.
- Therapy should be tailored to the individual with the use of fibrates, particularly gemfibrozil, and niacin for those individuals with elevated triglycerides.
- Caution should be exercised when using statins and fibrates in conjunction due to the high risk of rhabdomyolysis in later stages of CKD and this combination should generally be avoided in CKD stages 4 and 5.

Anaemia management in individuals with CKD has not been associated with a substantial improvement in outcomes.

- Current US Food and Drug Administration directives for anaemia treatment with epoetin suggest target haemoglobin levels of 10–12g/dL, based on data demonstrating a reduction in transfusions.
- No trial data has shown a survival benefit with anaemia treatment using epoetin or other erythropoiesis stimulating agents.

Despite the high risk of CVD, individuals with CKD are often undertreated.

- Less likely to receive aspirin, beta-blocking agents, ACEis, and lipid-lowering agents as well as revascularization therapies such as coronary artery bypass grafting and percutaneous angioplasty with stenting, following myocardial infarction despite suggestive evidence that these therapies are associated with improved survival regardless of the level of kidney function.

◆ In one of the few trials specifically targeting patients with kidney disease, a randomized controlled trial of fluvastatin 40mg daily increased to 80mg daily after two years vs placebo (ALERT), conducted in over 2,000 kidney transplant recipients, demonstrated a reduction in cardiac events but no reduction in mortality (Holdaas, et al., 2003). This is one of the few studies to show a definitive benefit to a primary study outcome in kidney disease and suggests that there likely is benefit to treating dyslipidaemia in individuals with reduced kidney function.

◆ Potential reasons for under-treatment include:

  • Minimal trial data on secondary prevention strategies in CKD providing quality evidence for treatment.

  • Therapeutic nihilism.

  • Justified and unjustified safety concerns.

Prevention and treatment of ischaemic heart disease: Stage 5 CKD/Dialysis

In **CKD stage 5/dialysis**, there are essentially no clinical trials demonstrating a significant survival benefit with any accepted coronary therapies in dialysis patients, leaving current practice decisions dependent on observational data and extrapolations from the non-CKD population. Whether this paucity of data has caused or is a consequence of a degree of therapeutic nihilism prevalent in the cardiac care of patients with advanced CKD is uncertain, but it, in part, reflects the fact that there are numerous competing causes of death in these patients and addressing only one at a time may not make a significant impact in reducing mortality.

Invasive management of ischaemic heart disease with angioplasty or bypass surgery is NOT contraindicated in dialysis patients.

◆ Several observational studies have shown that dialysis patients with coronary artery disease benefit from coronary revascularization and that, when appropriate, revascularization may be favourable to medical management.

BP management in dialysis patients presents unique challenges.

◆ Cohort studies are difficult to interpret as the highest BP are not associated with worse outcomes while there are graded increases in mortality with systolic BP <140mmHg.

- This altered risk factor pattern likely reflects limited cardiac reserve as well as reduced dietary intake in the individuals with the lowest BP.
- Proper assessment of BP is challenging in dialysis patients, particularly those on haemodialysis.
  - There are no data as to whether BP goals should reflect values before dialysis, after dialysis, or on days between dialysis.
  - Due to extensive arterial calcification and the presence of dialysis access (fistulas and grafts), it may be challenging to find a location to accurately measure BP.
- Opinion-based clinical practice guidelines, in the absence of solid observational or clinical trial evidence, have recommended a BP goal of <140/90mmHg pre-dialysis.
  - First accomplished by achieving appropriate dry weight (euvolaemia).
  - Pharmacologic therapy follows fluid management.
  - Avoidance of orthostatic and intradialytic hypotension is important in adjusting this BP goal upwards, if necessary.

Lipid, diabetes, diet, and lifestyle management are also challenging in dialysis patients due to the challenges of incorporating lifestyle changes, including diet and exercise, into an extremely regimented programme often requiring 15–20 hours weekly engaged in dialysis-related activities.

- Lipid management recommendations are summarized in Table 5.5 and focus primarily on patients with kidney failure requiring dialysis. Notably, these recommendations pre-date the completion of AURORA and the 4D trial discussed below as well as the ALERT trial discussed above; reflecting the overall paucity of trial data in dialysis, recommendations are based either on data of only moderate quality (B) or expert opinion (C). These are summarized in the bullets below.
  - Target serum LDL cholesterol <100mg/dL in individuals with known atherogenic disease.
  - No evidence to support this target given the results of the 4D trial, which compared atorvastatin to placebo in 1255 diabetic haemodialysis patients, and AURORA, which compared rosuvastatin to

placebo in haemodialysis patients age 50–80 years, with both studies revealing no benefit on a composite from cardiovascular causes, nonfatal myocardial infarction, or nonfatal stroke.

- Avoid the simultaneous use of statins and fibrates.
- Niacin use is safe in dialysis patients.

Table 5.5 Summary of Kidney Disease Outcome Quality Initiative (KDOQI) clinical practice guidelines for the assessment and management of dyslipidaemia in adult patients with CKD

Assessment	All patients with CKD should be evaluated for dyslipidaemias. (B)
	Assessment of dyslipidaemias should include a complete fasting lipid profile with total cholesterol, LDL, HDL, and triglycerides. (B)
	In dialysis patients, dyslipidaemias should be evaluated upon presentation (when the patient is stable), at 2–3 months after a change in treatment or other conditions known to cause dyslipidaemias, and at least annually thereafter. (B)
	In dialysis patients, a complete lipid profile should be measured after an overnight fast, whenever possible. (B)
	Haemodialysis patients should have lipid profiles measured either before dialysis or on days not receiving dialysis. (B)
	Dialysis patients with dyslipidaemias should be evaluated for remediable, secondary causes.* (B)
Treatment	In dialysis patients with fasting triglycerides >500mg/dL that cannot be corrected by removing an underlying cause, treatment with therapeutic lifestyle changes and a triglyceride-lowering agent should be considered. (C)
	In dialysis patients with LDL >100mg/dL, treatment should be considered to reduce LDL to <100mg/dL. (B)
	In dialysis patients with LDL <100mg/dL, fasting triglycerides >200mg/dL, and non-HDL cholesterol >130mg/dL, treatment should be considered to reduce non-HDL cholesterol to <130mg/dL. (C)

* Secondary causes include nephrotic syndrome, hypothyroidism, diabetes, excessive alcohol ingestion, chronic liver disease as well as medications, including highly active anti-retroviral therapy, beta-blockers, diuretics, androgens/anabolic steroids, oral contraceptives, corticosteroids, cyclosporine, and sirolimus; (B)=recommendation based on moderate clinical evidence that the practice will improve health outcomes; (C)=recommendation based on either weak evidence, poor evidence, or on the opinions of the Work Group and reviewers that the practice might improve net health outcomes.

To convert HDL, LDL, and total cholesterol from mg/dL to mmol/L, multiply by 0.026. To convert triglycerides to mmol/L, multiply by 0.011.

Glycaemia management:

- Reasonably tight diabetes control to a glycosylated haemoglobin level of <7% is likely reasonable in dialysis patients.

- Importantly, glycosylated haemoglobin levels may be unreliable in kidney failure, particularly in haemodialysis, reflecting the decreased survival time of red blood cells, and frequent glucose assessments should be included in a diabetes management plan.

- There may be a role for alternative measures of glucose control, including glycosylated albumin and fructosamine.

- In peritoneal dialysis, patients using icodextrin-based dialysate, finger stick assessments of glucose may be unreliable as icodextrin is metabolized to maltose.

  - Maltose cross-reacts with commonly used blood glucose monitoring systems, specifically those that use test strips containing the enzyme glucose dehydrogenase-pyrroloquinolinequinone or glucose dye oxidoreductase, and is interpreted as representing glucose.

  - This has resulted in hypoglycaemia following inappropriately high insulin doses and severe sequelae.

Diet and nutritional management:

- Challenging given the catabolic nature of the dialysis milieu and the frequent occurrence of protein-calorie malnutrition.

- Similar to other end-stage diseases, including heart failure and severe pulmonary diseases, obesity appears protective in dialysis patients.

- Obesity likely reflects a greater nutritional reserve.

  - Intentional weight loss for risk factor reduction, particularly in healthier dialysis patients, is likely to be beneficial.

  - Very difficult to accomplish given lifestyle and dietary limitations.

  - Potential role for bariatric surgery, particularly for potential kidney transplant recipients.

Smoking cessation in dialysis patients likely associated with improved survival.

Left ventricular hypertrophy (LVH) and heart failure

LVH and cardiomyopathy both occur as a consequence of atherosclerosis, arteriosclerosis, and CKD-associated risk factors, and may be exceedingly common in CKD because of the interplay among these risk factors (Table 5.6, Figure 5.4).

Epidemiology and pathophysiology of LVH and heart failure

Left ventricular hypertrophy is very common in individuals with CKD, far exceeding rates appreciated in the general population, with prevalence rates of approximately 30% in CKD stage 3 (GFR of

Table 5.6 Causes, risk factors, and manifestations of LVH and cardiomyopathy in CKD

Structural presentation	Notable risk factors	Indicators/ diagnostic test	Clinical sequelae
LVH	Pressure overload reflecting increased afterload due to hypertension, valvular disease, arteriosclerosis Volume overload reflecting volume retention due to progressive kidney disease ± anaemia	Echocardiography Cardiac magnetic resonance imaging Electrocardiography	Myocardial infarction Angina Sudden cardiac death Heart failure
Decreased LV contractility	Ischemic heart disease Hypertension LVH	Echocardiography	Cardiorenal syndrome Heart failure Myocardial infarction Angina Sudden cardiac death
Impaired LV relaxation	Hypertension Anaemia and volume overload Abnormal mineral metabolism Other arteriosclerosis risk factors LVH	Echocardiography	Heart failure Myocardial infarction Angina Sudden cardiac death

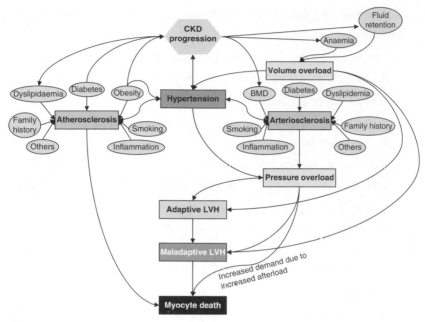

Fig. 5.4 Concept diagram representing a simplified overview of the relationship among CKD, kidney disease risk factors, CVD risk factors, and subsequent heart disease. Not all associations presented in this paradigm have been proven causal and for simplicity; not all connections are shown. BMD=bone and mineral disorder of CKD.

30–60mL/min/1.73m^2), 45% in stage 4 (GFR of 30–60mL/min/1.73m^2), and as high as 70% in incident dialysis patients.[19] Multiple factors in individuals with CKD may predispose to LVH and the interplay of these risk factors may subsequently lead to overt cardiomyopathy and heart failure.

LVH results from volume and pressure overload and it reflects an appropriate adaptation by the heart to these forces.

- With continued increased workload, the increased oxygen demands by the hypertrophied left ventricle exceed its perfusion, resulting in ischaemia and eventual myocyte death.

- In later stage CKD and dialysis patients, this inability to increase cardiac perfusion reflects not only LVH, but also the high prevalence of both atherosclerosis and arteriosclerosis limiting the ability of the vasculature to compensate for increased demand.

- Cardiomyopathy and heart failure may be the end result of this pathway.
  - Cardiomyopathy refers to the state of increased demand and decreased perfusion in the vast majority of CKD patients.
  - Additional contributors to the development of cardiomyopathy may include valvular disease and arrhythmias, both of which will be discussed later in this chapter.
  - Rare causes of cardiomyopathy in CKD include infiltrative diseases like amyloid and unusual sequelae of inflammatory diseases like lupus.

Incident and prevalent heart failure are also common in CKD, reflecting the development and progression of the factors predisposing to atherosclerosis, arteriosclerosis, and LVH in this population.

- CKD stages 3–4
  - Based on data from participants in the Atherosclerosis Risk In Communities (ARIC) study of community-dwelling residents age 45–64 years, those with eGFR <60mL/min/1.73m^2 at baseline were at twice the risk of being hospitalized for heart failure and death compared to participants with an eGFR of >90mL/min/1.73m^2, regardless of the presence of baseline coronary disease.
  - In a population of 60,000 insured individuals in Northern California diagnosed with chronic heart failure, 24% had an eGFR of 45–59mL/min/1.73m^2, 11% had an eGFR of 30–44mL/min/1.73m^2, and 4% had an eGFR <30mL/min/1.73m^2 (not receiving dialysis).
- CKD stage 5/dialysis
  - Approximately 25% of haemodialysis and 18% of peritoneal dialysis patients in the US will be diagnosed with heart failure annually.
  - Approximately 55% of prevalent haemodialysis patients are identified as having a history of heart failure.

Diagnosis of LVH and heart failure

In all stages of CKD, the diagnosis of LVH is readily accomplished with echocardiography, with cardiac function best assessed in the euvolaemic state as significant volume depletion and overload both reduce left ventricular inotropy.

♦ Two-dimensional echocardiogram results may be most meaningful on the interdialytic day as compared to immediately pre- or post-haemodialysis.

♦ Three-dimensional echocardiography may be useful to assess left ventricle (LV) structure as it avoids the use of geometric assumptions of LV shape that are required to estimate LV mass and volume.

♦ Magnetic resonance imaging may be more precise for assessing LV structure than echocardiography, but this technique is not yet widely available and the costs may be prohibitive.

♦ Despite no evidence supporting a benefit on outcomes, screening echocardiography is currently recommended for incident dialysis patients.

Treatment of LVH and heart failure

There are several potentially modifiable risk factors for LVH and heart failure that are highly prevalent in CKD patients, including anaemia, hypertension, extracellular volume overload, abnormal mineral metabolism (specifically hyperphosphataemia, secondary hyperparathyroidism, and vitamin D deficiency), and, on rare occasion, arteriovenous fistulae that cause high-output heart failure. Notably, in CKD patients, there is a paucity of trial data showing a definitive benefit of the modification of LVH risk factors for mortality outcomes, although there are substantial data on surrogate outcomes.

BP and volume management

♦ Two randomized, placebo-controlled trials studying individuals with diabetes and proteinuric CKD stages 3–4 have established a role for ARBs in reducing the risk of developing heart failure.

• No benefit in cardiovascular or all-cause mortality, probably reflecting insufficient power to evaluate these secondary outcomes.

♦ A recent, two-group, parallel, randomized controlled trial of 52 Canadian patients undergoing haemodialysis compared nocturnal haemodialysis six times weekly vs conventional haemodialysis three times weekly and noted an improvement in left ventricular mass in those undergoing frequent haemodialysis. This suggests that by reducing the volume and pressure overload that results in LVH, cardiac morphology may improve.

Anaemia management

• This has proven less conclusive for the treatment of LVH. Initial observational studies suggested that intensive anaemia management is associated with a regression in LV mass; however, this has not been borne out in clinical trials. Currently, some trial evidence suggests that partial correction of anaemia with epoetin may have beneficial effects on heart morphology, while normalization of anaemia likely offers no substantial benefit. The reasons for this are unclear, but may be related to potential adverse effects associated with high doses of epoetin.

• In Spanish patients with haemoglobin levels <10g/dL and a creatinine clearance of 10–40mL/min who participated in an open-label, non-randomized assessment of the effects of epoetin on heart morphology, there was a significant decrease in LV mass volume.

• In two randomized trials in CKD, targeting normalization or near-normalization of haemoglobin levels with epoetin had no effect on the surrogate outcome of LVH or LV mass index.

  • A Canadian trial, comparing haemoglobin targets of 12–14g/dL vs 9–10.5g/dL, showed no statistically significant difference between groups for the primary outcome of mean change in LV mass index; notably, BP was higher in the treatment group and the desired stratification between the lower and higher haemoglobin arms was not attained as the mean haemoglobin in the lower target group was 11.5g/dL.

  • A European trial, CREATE, randomized participants with CKD late stages 3 and 4 to receive treatment with epoetin to achieve target haemoglobin level of 13–15g/dL or to a target haemoglobin of 10.5–11.5g/dL, with or without epoetin therapy. They noted that the LV mass index did not significantly change within either group and that there was no significant difference between the two treatment groups in the final LV mass index.

Acute heart failure therapy

- This differs by CKD stage.
- In individuals with CKD not requiring dialysis, diuretics are the mainstay of therapy.
  - Recently, a role has been established for ultrafiltration, either with standard dialysis equipment or with a simpler apparatus that performs slow continuous ultrafiltration (SCUF) through more easily obtained vascular access.
  - Uncertain role for nesiritide (natriuretic peptide), which may have benefits in some patients, but overall has been associated with an increased progression to kidney failure.
- In dialysis patients, acute fluid overload is treated with ultrafiltration and may result either from heart failure or from marked fluid overload.
- In all stages of CKD, most recommendations for heart failure management are either extrapolated from the general population or are based on small trials, reflecting the paucity of quality studies.
  - ACEis and ARBs likely have both cardiac and kidney benefits independent of their BP-lowering effects in all CKD stages (Jafar, et al., 2003), including slowing the progression of kidney failure in individuals with proteinuria.
  - Aldosterone blockade may have further benefits. The utilization of aldosterone blockers like spironolactone may be limited by hyperkalaemia, especially when used in conjunction with ACEis and/or ARBs.
  - Beta-blocking agents, another mainstay of heart failure therapy in the general population, are also beneficial in patients with CKD. Reasonable evidence supports carvedilol use to reduce mortality risk in dialysis patients with LV dysfunction (Cice, et al., 2003). Atenolol should be avoided in advanced kidney disease due to the accumulation of toxic metabolites.

- Cardiac glycosides (e.g. digoxin) are frequently used in heart failure in the general population where they decrease morbidity but not mortality, but should be utilized judiciously, if at all, in advanced kidney disease, with careful attention to dosage, drug levels, and potassium balance.

Valvular and pericardial disease

Common valvular diseases in CKD include aortic and mitral valve stenosis and sclerosis as well as mitral annular calcification (Table 5.7). Endocarditis, a devastating complication that is particularly common in haemodialysis patients, is discussed elsewhere in this text.

- **In patients with CKD stages 3-4**, mitral valve calcification or mitral annular calcification was present in 20% of individuals with reduced kidney function (roughly CKD stages 3–4) in the Framingham Offspring study.
    - Independent statistically significant 60% increased odds of prevalent mitral annular calcification compared to those with an eGFR >60mL/min/1.73m^2.
    - Aortic valve calcification is also highly prevalent in individuals with CKD, but in studies like the Framingham Heart Study, this association is attenuated after adjustment for other risk factors.
- **In prevalent haemodialysis patients**, valvular disease becomes far more common.
    - 45% of subjects have calcification of the mitral valve and 34% of subjects have calcification of the aortic valve, compared with an expected prevalence of 3% to 5% in the general population.
    - Rates of mitral annular calcification range from 30–50% in haemodialysis patients.
- Disorders of mineral metabolism may predispose to valvular calcification in CKD.

Table 5.7 Causes, risk factors, and manifestations of valvular and pericardial disease in CKD

Disease type	Risk factors	Indicators/ diagnostic test	Clinical sequelae
Pericardial disease	Delayed or insufficient dialysis	Echocardiography	Heart failure Hypotension
Valvular disease	Bone and mineral disorder of CKD Aging Duration of dialysis	Echocardiography	Valvular stenosis Endocarditis Heart failure Arrhythmia Embolism
Mitral annular calcification	Bone and mineral disorder of CKD Other non-traditional risk factors?	Echocardiography reveals uniform, echodense, rigid band located near the base of posterior mitral leaflet	Arrhythmia Embolism Endocarditis Heart failure
Endocarditis	Valvular disease Chronic venous catheters	Echocardiography	Arrhythmia Heart failure Embolism

Arrhythmia and sudden cardiac death

All arrhythmias are extremely common in individuals with CKD, likely reflecting the high prevalence of ischaemic heart disease, structural heart disease, and electrolyte abnormalities.

Atrial fibrillation

- Prevalence estimates for paroxysmal and permanent atrial fibrillation are as high as 30% in dialysis patients (Abbott, et al., 2003).

- Of note, there are no trial data for the use of anti-arrhythmic agents in dialysis patients for rhythm control, although rhythm control has not been found to have significant advantages vs rate control in the general population.

- There are no trial data evaluating the use of warfarin to prevent embolic stroke in dialysis patients with atrial fibrillation.

- Theoretical advantages to chronic anticoagulation in dialysis patients with atrial fibrillation include the very high cardiovascular risk in these individuals as in the general population, individuals at the highest cardiovascular risk have had the greatest benefit with anticoagulation.
- Theoretical disadvantages to chronic anticoagulation in dialysis patients with atrial fibrillation include bleeding complications, specifically a high frequency of upper and lower gastrointestinal bleeds as well as a risk for intracerebral bleeds as haemodialysis patients have a greater fall risk, reflecting volume and blood pressure changes following the haemodialysis procedure.

Ventricular arrhythmias

Ventricular arrhythmias likely are exceedingly common although true rates cannot be determined.

- Prevalent dialysis patients have mortality rates of 62 deaths per 1,000 person years attributable to cardiac arrest (cause unknown) and arrhythmia (2003–2005 United States Renal Data System data).
- In the HEMO study of prevalent haemodialysis patients, death rates directly attributable to either arrhythmia or ischaemic heart disease (most commonly defined by sudden death in individual with prior coronary disease) were 51 per 1,000 person years.

There are few data on the prevention and treatment of arrhythmia and sudden cardiac death in the CKD population.

- Most current treatment recommendations mirroring those seen in the general population.
- The use of implantable cardioverter defibrillators (ICDs) in dialysis patients to reduce sudden cardiac death rates has been increasing exponentially over the past decade.
  - In 2005, 1,723 dialysis patients (0.6% of all dialysis patients) received an ICD.
  - ICD use has not been prospectively studied in the dialysis population and there have been no assessments of the cost to society per quality adjusted life year gained with this procedure.

Is cardiovascular disease a CKD risk factor?

This is a question that remains understudied. While renovascular disease can cause kidney disease, it is one of the less common causes of kidney failure, accounting for only 1.8% of incident dialysis patients. Severe heart failure can cause kidney disease secondary to decreased perfusion and systemic vasoconstriction (the cardiorenal syndrome) (Shlipak, et al., 2004), but the nature of the relationship between other ischaemic vascular disease and kidney disease is less well known. To date, there are a limited number of studies examining this question in generalizable populations. In an analysis of two US community-based cohorts, the presence of CVD increased the risk of a decline in kidney function sufficient to define an individual with CKD stage 3 by over 50% after adjusting for other traditional risk factors and demographic characteristics (Figure 5.5) (Elsayed, et al., 2007). Similar associations have been demonstrated in individuals with a clinical history of CVD and CKD stages 3–4 for progression to kidney failure.

Given these findings, several hypotheses remain:

- Kidney disease progression is caused by sequelae of ischaemic disease, whereby worsening cardiac function adds pre-renal factors to individuals with little functional kidney reserve.

- Ischaemic disease results in the addition of medications and interventions such as cardiac catheterization that may further exacerbate kidney injury.

- CKD and CVD are parallel manifestations of a single disease process, whereby a history of CVD may identify individuals with unrecognized, but subclinical or incipient kidney disease and a history of CKD may identify individuals with subclinical or incipient CVD.

Conclusions

CKD and CVD are commonly intertwined. The major risk factors for CKD, including older age, diabetes, and hypertension, are also the most important risk factors for CVD. Either reflecting shared comorbidity or perhaps reflecting a cycle by which kidney disease and CVD potentiate

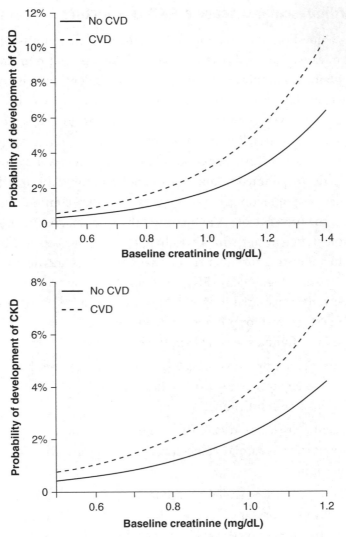

Fig. 5.5 Adjusted estimated probability of the development of kidney disease as a function of baseline estimated serum creatinine in (a) men and (b) women.

each other, individuals with CKD have an extremely high burden of co-existent CVD and are at high risk of manifesting subsequent CVD. Accordingly, there should be a high index of suspicion for cardiovascular complications in CKD, and, given the paucity of data guiding the diagnosis and treatment of CVD in CKD, far greater resources need to be devoted to the development and implementation of treatment strategies in this high-risk population.

References

Abbott, K.C., Trespalacios, F.C., Taylor, A.J., Agodoa, L.Y., 2003. Atrial fibrillation in chronic dialysis patients in the United states: risk factors for hospitalization and mortality. *BMC Nephrology*, 4(1), p.1.

Apple, F.S., Murakami, M.M., Pearce, L.A., Herzog, C.A., 2002. Predictive value of cardiac troponin I and T for subsequent death in end-stage renal disease. *Circulation*, 106(23), pp.2941–5.

Brosius, F.C. 3rd, Hostetter, T.H., Kelepouris, E., Mitsnefes, M.M., Moe, S.M., Moore, M.A., Pennathur, S., Smith, G.L., Wilson, P.W.; American Heart Association Kidney and Cardiovascular Disease Council; Council on High Blood Pressure Research; Council on Cardiovascular Disease in the Young; Council on Epidemiology and Prevention; Quality of Care and Outcomes Research Interdisciplinary Working Group, 2006. Detection of chronic kidney disease in patients with or at increased risk of cardiovascular disease: a science advisory from the American Heart Association Kidney And Cardiovascular Disease Council; the Councils on High Blood Pressure Research, Cardiovascular Disease in the Young, and Epidemiology and Prevention; and the Quality of Care and Outcomes Research Interdisciplinary Working Group: developed in collaboration with the National Kidney Foundation. *Circulation*, 114(10), pp.1083–7.

Cice G, Ferrara L, D'Andrea A, D'Isa, S., Di Benedetto, A., Cittadini, A., Russo, P.E., Golino, P., Calabro, R., 2003. Carvedilol increases two-year survivalin dialysis patients with dilated cardiomyopathy: a prospective, placebo-controlled trial. *Journal of the American College of Cardiology*, 41(9), pp.1438–44.

El-Abbadi, M., Giachelli, C.M., 2007. Mechanisms of vascular calcification. *Advances in Chronic Kidney Disease*, 14(1), pp.54–66.

Elsayed, E.F., Tighiouart, H., Griffith, J., Kurth, T., Levey, A.S., Salem, D., Sarnak, M.J., Weiner, D.E., 2007. Cardiovascular disease and subsequent kidney disease. *Archives of Internal Medicine*, 167(11), pp.1130–6.

Go, A.S., Chertow, G.M., Fan, D., McCulloch, C.E., Hsu, C.Y., 2004. Chronic kidney disease and the risks of death, cardiovascular events, and hospitalization. *New England Journal of Medicine*, 351(13), pp.1296–305.

Herzog, C.A., Ma, J.Z., Collins, A.J., 1998. Poor long-term survival after acute myocardial infarction among patients on long-term dialysis. *New England Journal of Medicine*, 339(12), pp.799–805.

Hillege, H.L., Fidler, V., Diercks, G.F., van Gilst, W.H., de Zeeuw, D., van Veldhuisen, D.J., Gans, R.O., Janssen, W.M., Grobbee, D.E., de Jong, P.E.; Prevention of Renal and Vascular End Stage Disease (PREVEND) Study Group, 2002. Urinary albumin excretion predicts cardiovascular and non-cardiovascular mortality in general population. *Circulation*, 106(14), pp.1777–82.

Himmelfarb, J., Stenvinkel, P., Ikizler, T.A., Hakim, R.M., 2002. The elephant in uremia: oxidant stress as a unifying concept of cardiovascular disease in uremia. *Kidney International*, 62(5), pp.1524–38.

Holdaas, H., Fellstrom, B., Jardine, A.G., Holme, I., Nyberg, G., Fauchald, P., Gronhagen–Riska, C., Madsen, S., Neumayer, H.H., Cole, E., Maes, B., Ambuhl, P., Olsson, A.G., Hartmann, A., Solbu, D.O., Pedersen, T.R.: Assessment of LEscol in Renal Transplantation (ALERT) Study Investigators, 2003. Effect of fluvastatin on cardiac outcomes in renal transplant recipients: a multicentre, randomised, placebo-controlled trial. *Lancet*, 361(9374), pp.2024–31.

Jafar, T.H., Stark, P.C., Schmid, C.H., Landa, M., Maschio, G., de Jong, P.E., de Zeeuw, D., Shahinfar, S., Toto, R., Levey, A.S.; AIPRD Study Group, 2003. Progression of chronic kidney disease: the role of blood pressure control, proteinuria, and angiotensin-converting enzyme inhibition: a patient-level meta-analysis. *Annals of Internal Medicine*, 139(4), pp.244–52.

Kalantar–Zadeh, K., Block, G., Humphreys, M.H., Kopple, J.D., 2003. Reverse epidemiology of cardiovascular risk factors in maintenance dialysis patients. *Kidney International*, 63(3), pp.793–808.

KDOQI, 2005. Clinical practice guidelines for cardiovascular disease in dialysis patients. *American Journal of Kidney Diseases*, 45(4 Suppl 3), S1–153.

Levin, A., Singer, J., Thompson, C.R., Ross, H., Lewis, M., 1996. Prevalent left ventricular hypertrophy in the predialysis population: identifying opportunities for intervention. *American Journal of Kidney Diseases*, 27(3), pp.347–54.

London, G.M., Marchais, S.J., Guerin, A.P., Metivier, F., 2002. Impairment of arterial function in chronic renal disease: prognostic impact and therapeutic approach. *Nephrology Dialysis Transplantation*, 17(Suppl 11), S13–5.

Ohtake, T., Kobayashi, S., Moriya, H., Negishi, K, Okamoto, K, Maesato, K, Saito, S., 2005. High prevalence of occult coronary artery stenosis in patients with chronic kidney disease at the initiation of renal replacement therapy: an angiographic examination. *Journal of the American Society of Nephrology*, 16(4), pp.1141–8.

Sarnak, M.J., Levey, A.S., 2000. Cardiovascular disease and chronic renal disease: a new paradigm. *American Journal of Kidney Diseases*, 35(4 Suppl 1), S117–31.

Sarnak, M.J., Levey, A.S., Schoolwerth, A.C., Coresh, J., Culleton, B., Hamm, L.L., McCullough, P.A., Kasiske, B.L., Kelepouris, E., Klag, M.J., Parfrey, P., Pfeffer, M., Raij, L., Spinosa, D.J., Wilson, P.W.; American Heart Association Councils on Kidney in Cardiovascular Disease, High Blood Pressure Research, Clinical Cardiology, and Epidemiology and Prevention, 2003. Kidney disease as a risk factor for development of cardiovascular disease: a statement from the American Heart Association Councils on Kidney in Cardiovascular Disease, High Blood Pressure Research, Clinical Cardiology, and Epidemiology and Prevention. *Circulation*, 108(17), pp.2154–69.

Shlipak, M.G., Massie, B.M., 2004. The clinical challenge of cardiorenal syndrome. *Circulation*, 110(12), pp.1514–7.

Strippoli, G.F., Navaneethan, S.D., Johnson, D.W., Perkovic, V., Pellegrini, F., Nicolucci, A., Craig, J.C., 2008. Effects of statins in patients with chronic kidney disease: meta-analysis and meta-regression of randomised controlled trials. *British Medical Journal*, 336(7645), pp.645–51.

Tonelli, M., Isles, C., Curhan, G.C., Tonkin, A., Pfeffer, M.A., Shepherd, J., Sacks, F.M., Furberg, C., Cobbe, S.M., Simes, J., Craven, T., West, M., 2004. Effect of pravastatin on cardiovascular events in people with chronic kidney disease. *Circulation*, 110(12), pp.1557–63.

Tonelli, M., Wiebe, N., Culleton, B., House, A., Rabbat, C., Fok, M., McAlister, F., Garg, A.X., 2006. Chronic kidney disease and mortality risk: a systematic review. *Journal of the American Society of Nephrology*, 17(7), pp.2034–47.

Weiner, D.E., Tabatabai, S., Tighiouart, H., Elsayed, E., Bansal, N., Griffith, J., Salem, D.N., Levey, A.S., Sarnak, M.J., 2006. Cardiovascular outcomes and all-cause mortality: exploring the interaction between CKD and cardiovascular disease. *American Journal of Kidney Diseases*, 48(3), pp.392–401.

Weiner, D.E., Tighiouart, H., Griffith, J.L., Elsayed, E., Levey, A.S., Salem, D.N., Sarnak, M.J., 2007. Kidney disease, Framingham risk scores, and cardiac and mortality outcomes. *American Journal of Medicine*, 120(6), pp.552 e1–8.

Chapter 6

Chronic kidney disease and infectious disease

Kar Neng Lai, Andrew S.H. Lai, and
Sydney C.W. Tang

Introduction

The pathogenetic links between infection and kidney disease are often
difficult to establish. The criteria for proving such causality are complex
and include, besides recognition of the clinical syndrome, the serological
diagnosis, identification of specific antigens related to the infective
organism, and the detection in glomerular/tubular structures of infective organism or its antigen(s) and host antibodies. According to Koch's
postulation, the aetiological link should be confirmed by complete cure
following eradication of the infective organism, an event that is, however, not always possible, especially in viral infection. In contrast to
acute bacterial infection, chronic viral infection is characterized by viral
antigens in higher concentrations in tissues than in the circulation,
where they are complexed with specific autoantibodies. Lately, viro-
logic and molecular analyses of pathologic tissues with the identification of the virus by techniques such as in situ hybridization, polymerase
chain reaction, and ultrastructural analysis have been successful in
demonstrating the presence of virus. Caution should be emphasized
that the tubular uptake of viral particles is common and does not
necessarily indicate an aetiological link of kidney disease. Improvement
of the kidney disease simultaneously with clearance of the suspected
antigen, or the recurrence of glomerulonephritis following re-infection,
provides additional clinical criteria.

Chronic kidney diseases (CKD) due to infection

Many forms of infection may be complicated by glomerulonephritis or interstitial nephritis although only a minority of patients will be involved. Some patients will develop CKD, especially when persistent infection occurs. Infection remains an important aetiology of CKD in the developing and under-developed countries. Table 6.1 lists infections known or reported to induce CKD. The most frequent and long recognized virus-related glomerulonephropathies are those associated with hepatitis B virus (HBV). Hepatitis C virus (HCV) in most cases is the aetiologic agent of cryoglobulinaemia-related mesangiocapillary glomerulonephritis. Human immunodeficiency virus (HIV) infection is related to a broad spectrum of glomerular involvement with multiple pathogenic mechanisms. This chapter focuses on CKD associated with common infection or infection with established aetiological links.

Mechanisms involved in the development of CKD associated with infection

Different mechanisms are operative in various infection-associated kidney diseases (Table 6.2). For acute glomerulonephritis, direct microbial infection of the glomerulus occurs with proliferative changes following the release of cytokines. In most cases, the nephropathy is reversible with rapid clearance of the organism. For the chronic form of glomerulonephritis, persistent infection providing a continuous antigenic stimulation, and hence resulting in antibody production and immune complexes formation, is essential. Earlier studies suggested the role of immune complexes (IC), derived from the circulation or formed in situ. Proteins derived from microbial organisms can cause inflammatory kidney diseases through the synthesis of various mediators that may cause sclerosis and worsen the glomerulopathy. A direct cytopathic effect of microbial proteins is also postulated. The other mechanism that operates in hepatitis C virus-induced mesangiocapillary glomerulonephritis (MCGN) is the induction of circulating cryoglobulins as an abnormal host response to infection. Cryoglobulins are either type II or type III, involving at least two classes of immunoglobulins, one of which is polyclonal in nature. In acute kidney injury associated with

Table 6.1 Infections leading to CKD

Bacterial	Chronic glomerulonephritis	Post-streptococcal glomerulonephritis
		Infective endocarditis
		Shunt nephritis
		Syphilis
	Interstitial nephritis	Leptospirosis
		Enteric fever
		Botryomycosis
		Legionella infection
Mycobacterial		Tuberculosis
		Leprosy
Viral	Chronic glomerulonephritis	HBV
		HCV
		HIV
		PV B19
	Interstitial nephritis	Hantavirus
		Polyoma virus BK
		Epstein–Barr virus
Protozoal		Amoebiasis
		Leishmaniasis (visceral)
		Malaria
		Schistosomiasis
		Dioctophymiasis (nematode infection)*
		Loiasis*
		Toxoplasmosis*
Fungal		Candidiasis
		Aspergillosis
Miscellaneous	(Chronic infective inflammation)	Reflux nephropathy
		Xanthogranulomatous pyelonephritis
		Malacoplakia
		Megalocytic interstitial nephritis

* Mechanism and pathology not well defined

Table 6.2 Mechanisms of kidney injury induced by infective agents

Circulating IC involving:

Antigen(s) derived from the infective organism and host-specific antibodies

Endogenous antigens modified by injury induced by the organism and host auto-antibodies

In situ immune-mediated mechanisms involving antigen(s) derived from the infective organism bound to glomerular structures

Expression of protein(s) derived from the infective organism or abnormal host proteins in tissue, inducing:

Cell death through necrosis, or apoptosis, or cell dysfunction

Increased matrix synthesis and/or decreased matrix degradation

Release of cytokines, chemokines, and adhesion molecules, growth factors

Direct cytopathogenic effect on glomerular cells with undefined mechanisms

Tubulointerstitial injuries either due to direct cytopathogenic effect or secondary to mediators released by glomerular inflammation

Direct destructive effect of the invasive microbial(s)

Fibrotic replacement of normal kidney tissue secondary to healing

Haemodynamic disturbance, multi-organ failure

Complicating rhabdomyolysis, hepatorenal syndrome

Nephrotoxicity of anti-microbial therapy (occasional)

---

hantavirus or SARS-coronavirus infection, the pathogenetic mechanisms of interstitial nephritis, disseminated intravascular coagulopathy, and multi-organ failure are predominant culprits instead of IC formation.

Bacterial glomerulopathy

Post-streptococcal glomerulonephritis (PSGN)

Pathogenesis

- Acute nephritis related to group A (beta-haemolytic) streptococci, commonly type 12.

- The nephritogenic factor in group A streptococci may be only loosely linked to M protein type.

- The pathology is characterized by diffuse endocapillary proliferative glomerulonephritis with polymorph exudation and IgG and C3 deposits.

- Only rarely co-exists with rheumatic fever.

Clinical features

- Principally a disease of children and usually presents as acute nephritic syndrome.

- The diagnosis is characterized by raised anti-streptolysin O titre, low serum complement 3, and positive throat culture for group A beta-haemolytic streptococci; a kidney biopsy usually is not required.

- The incidence falls drastically in developed countries, probably related to less virulent streptococcal infection and the frequent use of antibiotics.

Course and prognosis

- The immediate prognosis for acute PSGN is favourable with supportive treatment, including antibiotics.

- The majority of paediatric patients with well-documented, sporadic or epidemic acute PSGN have good long-term prognosis if there is no evidence of pre-existing kidney disease, persistent heavy proteinuria, or extensive crescentic glomerular lesions at the onset.

- The long-term prognosis of adult PSGN may not be totally favourable, especially in the elderly.

- The development of histological and clinical 'chronicity' after acute glomerulonephritis occurs in 8–20% of patients, with high risk in blacks of Puerto Rican extraction, and those with heavy proteinuria and hypertension at the onset.

- The progression to end-stage renal failure (ESRF) was documented in several instances.

- Recurrence of true PSGN is uncommon.

Infective endocarditis

Pathogenesis

- In the present antimicrobial era, glomerulonephritis appears among patients who present late for treatment and in whom the site of valvular abnormality may not be obvious.

- More frequently, this disorder is observed among heroin addicts with right-sided endocarditis and negative blood culture results.

- Immune-mediated pathology supported by circulating immune complexes (CIC), glomerular IgG, IgM, and C3, and detection of bacterial antigens in glomerular IC.
- The pathology is characterized by focal and segmental, proliferative, glomerular lesions, sometimes with focal fibrinoid necrosis or capillary thrombi.

Clinical features

- Variable clinical manifestations with acute or subacute onset and involvement in any heart valves: microscopic or gross haematuria, nephrotic syndrome (25%), and incidental finding of raised serum creatinine. Cardiac murmur may be absent in right-sided endocarditis.
- Late and inadequate antimicrobial treatment may lead to CKD or irreversible kidney failure.
- Cardiac assessment for valvular function and opinion for valvular surgery should be part of the management strategy.

Shunt nephritis

Pathogenesis

- Complication following colonization of body shunts with microorganisms.
- More frequent in ventriculo-vascular shunt (up to 27%) followed by ventriculo-atrial shunt. Ventriculo-peritoneal shunts are more resistant to infection.
- The pathology is characterized by mesangial proliferative or mesangiocapillary (type 1) glomerulonephritis with diffuse granular and capillary IgG, IgM, and C3 deposits.
- Infecting bacterial antigens have been identified in glomerular deposits.

Clinical features

- Variable clinical manifestations: most commonly fever (84%), microscopic or gross haematuria, moderate or nephrotic range proteinuria (30%), azotaemia, anaemia, hepatosplenomegaly, purpura, arthralgia, and adenopathy.

- Laboratory investigation shows hypocomplementaemia, rheumatoid factor, cryoglobulin, CIC, and elevated C-reactive protein.

Course and prognosis

- Early recognition and prompt antimicrobial therapy together with shunt removal lead to clinical healing of the glomerular lesions in most instances.
- In some patients, glomerulonephritis does not resolve for several years after elimination of the infective organism or stimulus.
- Persistent kidney insufficiency marked by proteinuria and haematuria occurs in one third of cases although hypertension is not common.
- Progression to ESRF has been reported.

Syphilis

Pathogenesis

- Glomerular pathology complicates congenital or acquired (secondary-stage) syphilis.
- Glomerulonephritis is a well-established, but rather uncommon complication of congenital or latent secondary syphilis. Regardless of the clinical course and histological type, these patients were all characterized by strongly positive results of serologic tests for syphilis.
- The typical pathology is membranous nephropathy although minimal change disease and rapidly progressive glomerulonephritis have also been reported. In membranous nephropathy, treponemal antigen is detected in the subepithelial area of the glomerular basement membrane.

Clinical features

- The most common kidney manifestations are proteinuria and nephrotic syndrome. Microscopic haematuria may be occasionally present. Acute kidney injury is a rare and exceptional presentation.
- Anti-syphilitic therapy is the treatment of choice with excellent results, though on occasion, the resolution of nephrotic syndrome may take months.
- Chronic kidney insufficiency has been documented in patients with latent syphilitic nephropathy.

Bacterial interstitial nephritis

Leptospirosis

◆ Kidney involvement is common in leptospirosis. Leptospiral infection is characterized by the diagnostic triad of fever, icterus, and acute kidney injury. Acute kidney injury is observed in 44–67% of patients. Clinical manifestations vary from urinary sediment changes to acute kidney injury. Severe hypotension is an important warning sign for the later development of cardiopulmonary, haemorrhagic, and kidney complications.

◆ Interstitial nephritis is the basic kidney lesion. Vasculitis is observed in the acute phase of the disease. Tubular necrosis and interstitial nephritis are responsible for kidney failure. Glomerular changes usually are not remarkable.

◆ Convalescents recovered from acute icterohaemorrhagic leptospirosis may also develop slowly regressing kidney dysfunctions, most frequent of which are chronic kidney disease, pyelonephritis and tubulointerstitial nephritis, and arterial hypertension. Kidney disorders may be due to immunopathological reactions followed by the activation of bacterial microflora.

◆ Interestingly, in bovine leptospirosis, kidney damage is not so severe, but it tends to progress.

Legionnaires' disease

◆ *Legionella pneumophila* grows well in water up to 40°C in temperature and the infection is almost certainly spread by aerosol route. Pneumonia is the main presentation. Occasionally, haematuria occurs with kidney failure.

◆ Acute kidney injury complicating *Legionella* infection is associated with acute tubulointerstitial nephritis, acute tubular necrosis, rhabdomyolysis, or rapidly progressive crescentic glomerulonephritis.

◆ Occasionally, chronic kidney disease develops in patients with *Legionella* infection despite successfully treated for pneumonia. The chronic kidney disease can be the sequel of rapidly progressive crescentic glomerulonephritis, progression from acute to chronic interstitial nephritis, and rarely, chronic interstitial nephritis in the absence of pulmonary signs or symptoms. In the last instance, manifestations of kidney involvement include proteinuria, haematuria, pyuria, cylindruria, and azotaemia. A toxic metabolite produced by *Legionella pneumophila* has been theorized to produce a vasoconstrictive effect on the kidney microvasculature, leading to ischaemia and kidney dysfunction.

Enteric fever

- Salmonella infection is typified by acute kidney injury secondary to acute interstitial nephritis, rhabdomyolysis, or multi-organ failure.

- In areas endemic for hepatosplenic schistosomiasis, prolonged Salmonella bacteraemia exacerbates a pre-existing, subclinical schistosomal glomerulopathy, commonly presented as nephrotic syndrome or significant proteinuria.

Botryomycosis

- Botryomycosis is a rare, inflammatory, chronic, suppurative, bacterial infection that presents as a slow-growing, soft tissue mass with a purulent discharge, and closely mimics fungal infections, both clinically and histologically. It is usually caused by chronic, low–grade bacterial infections. The causative organisms are *Staphylococcus aureus* and *Pseudomonas aeruginosa*. The condition has two forms; cutaneous or disseminated visceral, and the latter has a poor prognosis.

- Kidney botryomycosis is not uncommonly mistaken for a kidney carcinoma in the clinical setting of a kidney mass. The lesion is composed of confluent abscesses containing 'sulphur, granule-like' lesions in which irregularly lobed aggregates of Gram-negative organisms are surrounded by an eosinophilic capsule.

- In histological study, botryomycosis is difficult to differentiate from actinomycosis and mycosis. Therefore, histochemical stains are necessary to make the differential diagnosis.

+ The disease is known to develop in immunocompetent patients. However, impaired phagocytosis due to other medical illness (e.g. diabetes mellitus) may be contributory to the susceptibility.

Mycobacterial infection

Tuberculosis

Pathogenesis

+ Infection predominantly caused by the human tubercle bacillus, *Mycobacterium tuberculosis*, but *Mycobacterium bovis* occasionally can be responsible.

+ Approximately 10% of new cases of tuberculosis reported annually are extrapulmonary and the genitourinary tract is the leading site.

+ Can affect the kidney insidiously with azotaemia and smooth, equal-sized kidneys on imaging. Pathology is characterized by chronic tubulointerstitial nephritis with granuloma formation.

+ Chronic tuberculosis sometimes is complicated by amyloidosis, papillary necrosis, and hypercalcaemia.

+ Genitourinary tuberculosis usually results from 'silent' bacillaemia accompanying pulmonary tuberculosis. Spread to the kidney pelvis produces a tuberculous pyelonephritis that may even progress to a pyonephrosis-like lesion, also known as a 'cement' or 'putty' kidney. Scarring develops within the kidney pelvis with calcification in 24% of cases, identifiable as kidney or ureteric stones in up to 19% of cases. Infection frequently spreads down the ureters into the bladder, producing mucosal and mural granulomatous lesions associated with scarring. The clinical consequences of an extensive kidney lesion include autonephrectomy. The destructive kidney lesions may spread outside the kidney capsule and produce a mass lesion, which can mimic a neoplasm. Ureteric involvement also may produce irregular ureteric strictures and segmental dilation, leading to obstruction and/or reflux. Keratinizing squamous metaplasia may develop as a late complication of chronic inflammation and infection of the kidney pelvis, and may persist even after treatment of the active tuberculous lesion. This is a potential risk factor for the development of squamous carcinoma in chronic cases.

Clinical and laboratory findings

- Many patients present with lower urinary symptoms typical of 'conventional' bacterial cystitis, and suspicions of tuberculosis are aroused when urine examination reveals unexplained 'sterile' pyuria. Other symptoms that sometimes occur include back, flank and suprapubic pain, haematuria, frequency, and nocturia; these might also suggest conventional bacterial urinary tract infection. Kidney colic is uncommon (<10%) and constitutional symptoms also are unusual. Only one third of patients have an abnormal chest X-ray.

- Diagnosed by acid-fast bacilli by microscopy and/or culture, nucleic acid amplification techniques for *Mycobacterium tuberculosis*.

Treatment

- Modern short-course anti-tuberculosis drug regimens are effective in all forms of tuberculosis. They are based on an initial 2-month intensive phase of treatment in which usually, four drugs—rifampicin, isoniazid, pyrazinamide, and ethambutol (or streptomycin)—are given. This is followed by a 4-month continuation phase in which only rifampicin and isoniazid are given, with the aim of eliminating the few remaining near-dormant, persisting bacilli. For success, all doses must be taken and drug compliance is essential.

- Recently, there has been a worrying increase in the incidence of multidrug-resistant tuberculosis which, by definition, is caused by bacilli resistant to rifampicin and isoniazid, with or without resistance to other drugs. Therapy requires the use of at least four drugs that are selected on the basis of drug susceptibility tests, from ethionamide, prothionamide, quinolones (e.g. ofloxacin), newer macrolides (e.g. clarithromycin), cycloserine, kanamycin, viomycin, capreomycin, thiacetazone, and para-amino-salicylic acid. These are less effective and the duration of therapy is based on bacteriologic response, but may be 18 months or longer.

- Special considerations apply to the treatment of tuberculosis in patients with impaired kidney function.

- Surgical intervention is indicated in cases of advanced unilateral disease complicated by pain or haemorrhage and for bladder augmentation. Surgical excision of non-functioning kidneys or extensive lesions in partly functioning kidneys is controversial. Relief of ureteric obstruction by stenting or percutaneous nephrostomy may aid functional recovery, especially in patients with good kidney cortical thickness, limited kidney involvement, and a GFR of more than 15mL/min.

Leprosy

Pathogenesis

+ Infection caused by *Mycobacterium leprae*, more common with erythema nodosum leprosum.

+ The frequency of glomerulonephritis complicating leprosy varies from 6 to 63%, probably due to patient selection.

+ Glomerular pathologies include mesangiocapillary glomerulonephritis (type 1), mesangial proliferative glomerulonephritis, and endocapillary proliferative glomerulonephritis. Occasionally, oliguric, acute kidney injury can occur with the development of crescentic glomerulonephritis. Immunofluorescence study suggests IC-mediated pathology.

+ Other kidney pathologies include chronic interstitial nephritis, nephrosclerosis, granulomas, and amyloidosis. Amyloidosis is more frequently associated with lepromatous leprosy with recurrent bouts of erythema nodosum leprosum.

Clinical course

+ Microscopic haematuria and proteinuria are key features of glomerulonephritis.

+ Glomerulonephritis, interstitial nephritis, and amyloidosis all lead to chronic kidney disease and ESRF. Amyloidosis is associated with heavy proteinuria and carries a high mortality.

+ A high index of suspicion for 'renal leprosy' in endemic areas (Brazil, India, and Madagascar) and in azotaemic patients with skin rash/pigmentation.

+ Kidney impairment may also be a complication of treatment for leprosy (dapsone, rifampicin, and clofazimine).

Viral glomerulopathy

HBV-associated glomerulonephritis

Virology

- HBV is a hepatotropic, double-stranded deoxyribonucleic acid (DNA) virus of the Hepadnaviridae family.

- HBV is itself not cytopathic; hepatitis develops as a result of the host's immune reaction towards infected hepatocytes. HBV utilizes a replication strategy closely related to retroviruses in that transcription of RNA into DNA is a critical step. Unlike retroviruses, HBV DNA is not integrated into host cell DNA during replication. After an HBV particle binds to and enters a hepatocyte, HBV DNA enters the cell nucleus and is converted into covalently closed, circular DNA which is highly stable, acting as the intermediate template for transcription of RNA copies. This pre-genomic messenger ribonucleic acid (mRNA) is transported to the cytoplasm, and has the dual functions of acting as a template for the synthesis of new HBV DNA and carrying genetic information to direct the synthesis of viral proteins

- Today, an estimated 350–400 million people worldwide are infected with HBV. In endemic areas, transmission is usually vertical from infected mother to child. Horizontal transmission occurs via direct contact with blood (as in blood transfusions), or mucous membranes (as in sexual contacts), or via the percutaneous route upon contact with blood or body fluids (as in intravenous drug use and needle-sharing practices).

Pathogenesis

- The three main glomerulonephritis associated with HBV infection are membranous nephropathy (MN), mesangiocapillary glomerulonephritis (MCGN) and IgA nephropathy (IgAN).

- MN is more frequently reported in Asian populations and in paediatric cases. The diagnosis of HBV-associated glomerulonephritis in most reports was based on the following criteria: the persistent presence of circulating HBV antigen or HBV DNA, no other causes of glomerulonephritis, and the presence of HBV-specific antigen(s) or viral genome in the glomerulus. In clinical practice, regression of the pathology with viral eradication is not easily demonstrable because of ethical concerns to repeat kidney biopsies in human subjects after clinical remission. Hence, the diagnosis of HBV-associated kidney disease in reality relies heavily upon the demonstration of HBV-specific antigen(s) in the glomeruli.

• The role of HBV as an aetiological agent is supported by animal studies in woodchucks and demonstration of HBV antigens (HBsAg for IgAN and HBeAg for MN and MCGN) in the human glomerulus by molecular technique.

Clinical findings

• Paediatric and adult patients tend to have slightly different clinical manifestations of HBV-related MN.

• In children, there is a strong male preponderance, and the most frequent presentation is nephrotic syndrome together with microscopic haematuria and normal or mildly impaired kidney function. Paediatric chronic HBV carriers often do not have overt liver disease and transaminase levels are usually normal.

• In adults, proteinuria or nephrotic syndrome are the most common manifestations, though a male predominance is less obvious than that observed in children. In addition, adults are more likely than children to have hypertension, kidney dysfunction, and clinical evidence of liver disease.

• The prognosis of HBV-associated MN in children is favourable with stable kidney function and high rates of spontaneous remission reported in several high prevalence areas. On the other hand, adults with HBV-associated MN typically develop progressive disease. In endemic area, up to 29% of patients had progressive kidney failure and another 10% developed terminal uraemia over five years.

• The prognosis is even worse in patients with nephrotic range proteinuria and overt hepatitis at presentation, with over 50% of patients requiring renal replacement therapy (RRT) over three years. Prognosis is worse in those with vertical versus those with horizontal transmission and also worse in endemic versus sporadic infection.

- Apart from MN, other kidney pathologies have also been reported in association with HBV infection. These include MCGN with or without cryoglobulinaemia, mesangial proliferative glomerulonephritis, and IgAN.

- Occasionally, overlapping of these pathologic forms may lead to double glomerulopathies. For instance, MN and IgAN have been reported to co-exist in a HBV carrier.

Laboratory findings

- Kidney biopsy shows capillary deposits of HBeAg in MN and MCGN, and mesangial deposits of HBsAg in IgAN.

- Diagnostic and therapeutic assessments include standard liver biochemistry (serum alanine aminotransferase, γ-glutamyltransferase, and bilirubin levels), and HBV serologies (HBsAg, HBeAg, anti-HBe, and anti-HBc antibodies).

- Subjects with biochemical hepatitis should also be tested for circulating HBV DNA levels and undergo liver biopsy. In addition, α-fetoprotein assay could be an important adjunct. Serum C3 and C4 levels may be low in 20–50% of patients.

Clinical approach

- Unlike childhood disease with a high rate of spontaneous remission, adults with HBV-associated MN typically develop progressive disease.

- Treatment for HBV-associated kidney disease should ideally achieve the following objectives: (i) amelioration of nephrotic syndrome and its complications, (ii) preservation of kidney function, (iii) normalization of liver function and prevention of hepatic complications of HBV, and (iv) permanent eradication of HBV.

- In view of the IC nature of the disease, immunosuppressive therapy, similar to that applied in the idiopathic form of the disease, was once fashionable.

- Although corticosteroid has been previously reported to achieve symptomatic relief in isolated cases, the contemporary view is that steroid and cytotoxic agents may cause deleterious hepatic flares or even fatal decompensation by enhancing viral replication upon treatment withdrawal.

Treatment

- Interferon-α is a naturally occurring cytokine that possesses anti-viral, anti-proliferative, and immunomodulatory effects. While reported to be useful in children, interferon-α has produced mixed results in adults with HBV-associated MN.

- A nucleoside analogue, lamivudine (−) enantiomer of 3'-thiacytidine, inhibits DNA synthesis by terminating the nascent, pro-viral DNA chain through interference with the reverse transcriptase activity of HBV. In children and adults with HBV-associated MN, lamivudine has been reported in case reports and uncontrolled trials to induce remission of nephrotic syndrome and suppress viral replication. A potential limitation of prolonged treatment with lamivudine is the emergence of drug-resistant strains (10% per year) due to the induction and selection of HBV variants with mutations at the YMDD motif of DNA polymerase.

- Two agents that might be considered in case of lamivudine resistance are adefovir dipivoxil and entecavir. The former is an acyclic nucleotide analogue which is effective against both lamivudine-resistant HBV mutants as well as wild type HBV. The latter is a deoxyguanine nucleoside analogue effective for active viral replication or histologically active disease. Entecavir has demonstrated greater suppression of viral replication compared with lamivudine. Entecavir can be used either as a primary therapeutic agent or for HBV-hepatitis of lamivudine resistance.

- Both agents are potentially nephrotoxic and dose adjustment is needed according to kidney function. There is no randomized clinical trial on its efficacy in HBV-related GN.

Prevention

- Short of an ideal agent for the treatment of HBV-associated glomerulopathy, active immunization remains the most effective measure of immunoprophylaxis. The introduction of active immunization to all newborns in Taiwan, Hong Kong, and the US has led to a dramatic (10-fold) decline in the incidence of neonatal HBV infection and its subsequent sequelae.

* In 2003, the World Health Organization recommended that all countries provide universal HBV immunization programmes for infants and adolescents.

HCV-associated glomerulonephritis

Virology

* HCV is a small RNA virus in the Flaviridae family that has evolved into six genotypes with more than 50 subtypes.

* Two immunologic features predispose to extrahepatic disease manifestations: (i) the evasion of immune elimination, leading to chronic infection and the accumulation of CIC, and (ii) the production of monoclonal rheumatoid factors (RF), causing type II cryoglobulinaemia and related vasculitis.

* The prevalence of mixed cryoglobulinaemia increases with the duration of the hepatitis. HCV carriers have high prevalence of mixed cryoglobulinaemia (35–90%). Frank symptomatic cryoglobulinaemia occurs in 1% or less of patients and usually is associated with high levels of RF and cryoglobulins. Testing unselected patients with cryoglobulinaemia has shown that up to 90% have anti-HCV antibody.

* To date, around 170–200 million individuals worldwide are estimated to have chronic HCV infection. The transmission is horizontal through body fluid.

Pathogenesis

* The principal kidney manifestation of HCV infection is MCGN type I, usually in the context of cryoglobulinaemia.

* MCGN associated with type II cryoglobulinaemia is the predominant type of glomerulonephritis clinically associated with HCV infection. The prevalence of MCGN in HCV type II cryoglobulinaemia is approximately 30%. MCGN also is occasionally observed in patients with hepatitis C in the absence of cryoglobulinaemia.

Clinical findings

* Kidney disease is rare in children and the typical age of disease onset is in the fifth or sixth decade of life after long-standing infection,

often in association with mild subclinical liver disease. Other symptoms of cryoglobulinaemia such as palpable purpura and arthralgias may occur.

◆ Kidney manifestations include nephrotic (20%) or non-nephrotic proteinuria and microhaematuria. Acute nephritic syndrome occurs in 25% of cases. Progression to uraemia is associated with male gender and old age. Kidney insufficiency, frequently mild, occurs in about half of the patients. The clinical course can vary dramatically. The kidney disease tends to have an indolent course and does not progress to uraemia despite the persistence of urinary abnormalities in the majority of patients. Around 15% of patients eventually require dialysis according to an Italian series. MN is the other form of glomerular lesion in HCV carriers and is characterized by the absence of cryoglobulin and a male predominance.

◆ Over 80% of patients have refractory hypertension responsible for a considerable number of cardiovascular deaths.

Laboratory findings

◆ Laboratory testing coupled with kidney biopsy establishes the diagnosis of HCV-related MCGN.

◆ Most patients will have anti-HCV antibody as well as HCV RNA in serum.

◆ Serum transaminase levels are elevated in 70% of patients. Cryoglobulins are detected in 50–70% of patients. Serum electrophoresis and immunofixation reveals type II mixed cryoblobulins in which the monoclonal RF, almost invariably an IgMκ, is a distinguishing feature of cryoglobulinaemic glomerulonephritis.

◆ Urine κ light chains are also commonly present.

◆ The serum complement pattern, which does not change much with clinical activity, is also discriminative. Characteristically, the early complement components (C4 and C1q) and CH50 are at very low, or even undetectable, levels while C3 levels tend to remain normal or only slightly depressed.

Treatment

- In general, therapy can be directed at two levels: (1) the removal of cryoglobulins by plasmapheresis; and (2) the inhibition of their synthesis through either attenuation of the immune responses (using steroid or cytotoxic agents) or suppression of viral replication (using interferon and ribavirin).

- Controlled trials have shown that anti-viral therapy with interferon-α is associated with improvements in systemic symptoms of IC disease. However, a relapse after therapy occurs in a large proportion of patients, particularly with interferon monotherapy given for short durations. Combination therapy with interferon-α2b plus ribavirin represented an important milestone for the treatment of chronic hepatitis C infection.

- The introduction of pegylated forms of interferon (peginterferon) and the subsequent combination with ribavirin in treating HCV infection are encouraging. This is also effective in HCV-associated cryoglobulinaemic MCGN. One therapeutic drawback lies in the haemolytic effect complicating ribavirin therapy, particularly in patients with functional kidney impairment. This therapeutic difficulty has been overcome by adjusting the dose according to the glomerular filtration rate instead of body weight alone and utilizing recombinant erythropoietin to overcome anaemia.

- A higher treatment failure rate of HCV carriers with genotype 1 is recognized.

- Preliminary studies with rituximab therapy of HCV-related cryoglobulinaemic glomerulonephritis have given encouraging results, even if a point of caution is important, because rituximab use may be associated with the activation of various infections, including HCV.

HIV-related glomerular diseases

- Table 6.3 summarizes the clinicopathological features of the wide spectrum of glomerulopathies occurring in the course of HIV infection.

Table 6.3 Different spectrum of glomerulonephritis complicating HIV infection

Disease entity	Pathology	Clinical features	Progression to ESRF
Classical HIV-associated nephropathy (HIV-AN)	Focal segmental glomerulosclerosis (FSGS) with tuft collapse or, more rarely, mesangial hyperplasia, likely a direct effect of HIV or viral proteins on the kidney epithelium. Glomerular changes are capillary wall collapse of various severities, with widening of Bowman's space. Visceral epithelial cells show hyperplasia and hypertrophy, with protein inclusions in their swollen cytoplasm, surrounding the collapsed lobules. Sclerosis involves segments of capillary tuft or diffusely the whole glomerular surface. Tubular cells may present degenerative changes, necrosis, or flattening, with large dense casts in dilated tubules. Detection of HIV RNA and DNA in tubular and glomerular epithelial cells suggests direct infection. In addition, kidney uptake of viral gene products may induce transactivation of host genes. HIV proteins affect kidney cells in their biological response in various ways: apoptosis, phenotypic modifications, and subsequently tubulointerstitial fibrosis.	Most common (10%) of all HIV-infected patients, mainly males with risk of drug abuse and often affects African American. Clinical manifestations are nephrotic range proteinuria and kidney insufficiency. Hypertension and oedema are uncommon. By ultrasonography, in overt cases, patients typically have enlarged, highly echogenic kidneys, probably related to microcystic tubular dilatation.	Before effective anti-retroviral treatment, it ran a rapid, downhill, clinical course. Intensive anti-retroviral treatment exerts a beneficial effect in delaying the progression.

Table 6.3 (Continued) Different spectrum of glomerulonephritis complicating HIV infection

Disease entity	Pathology	Clinical features	Progression to ESRF
HIV IC-mediated disease	Diffuse proliferative-mesangiocapillary or lupus-like glomerulonephritis, with parietal immune deposits. Viral antigen was detected in glomeruli and antibodies eluted from the kidney reacted with HIV antigens present in CIC. These complexes were IgA-p24 antigen, IgG-p24, and IgG-gp120. In cases of HIV-related IgAN, circulating IC containing IgA idiotype antibodies are detected.	Nephrotic syndrome with microscopic haematuria. Patients often have HCV co-infection, but HIV seems to have the prevailing role.	Progression to kidney failure, but more slowly than HIV-AN. In HIV-related IgAN, the progression to kidney failure is more rapid than non-HIV cases.
Heterogeneous pathologies	Heterogeneous histologies; one example is immunotactoid glomerulonephritis; the role of HIV infection is uncertain.		Yes
HIV-associated thrombotic microangiopathy/ haemolytic uraemic syndrome	Thrombotic microangiopathy/haemolytic uraemic syndrome	Acute kidney injury, microscopic haematuria, and non-nephrotic proteinuria. Multi-organ involvement is frequent, and the prognosis is bad, with a high rate of mortality. Multifactorial aetiologies, including drug, neoplasia, lymphoma, or infection may be operative.	Yes

- Ethnic-geographic background is an important feature, with a high prevalence of African and African American origin in collapsing FSGS .

- ESRF due to HIV-associated nephropathy (HIV-AN) is 12 times more likely to occur in African Americans than in whites.

- Progression to ESRF in patients with proven HIV-AN is reduced with the use of a highly active antiretroviral therapy compared with a nucleoside analogue (zidovudine). Both are superior to no treatment.

Parvovirus B19 (PV B19)

- PV B19 has been associated with acute glomerulonephritis with its pathology characterized by endocapillary and/or MCGN with sub-endothelial deposits. Spontaneous recovery is the usual clinical course.

- PV B19 can also be associated with collapsing glomerulopathy. A significantly higher prevalence of PV B19 DNA has been detected in kidney biopsies (78%) and in peripheral blood (87%) from patients affected by collapsing glomerulopathy, compared with other nephropathies.

- The glomerular and tubular infection by PV B19 may trigger collapsing glomerulopathy, but only in patients with immune defects and with a racial predisposition (African).

Viral interstitial nephritis

Hantavirus

- An enveloped, single-stranded RNA virus belonging to the family Bunyaviridae which is maintained in specific insectivores or rodent host species. Transmission to humans occurs via direct contact with faeces, urine, and saliva of infected rodents, in particular, by inhaling virus-contaminated aerosol.

- Normally, hantaviruses are responsible for 'haemorrhagic fever with renal syndrome', an acute interstitial nephritis due to direct vascular injury in kidney tissue. The severe form leads to acute kidney injury in 50% of the cases while the less severe forms occur in non-endemic areas, mainly presenting with fever, hepatitis, and mild kidney impairment.

◆ Its role in the development of chronic kidney failure has been suggested by the higher incidence of antibodies to hantavirus not only in endemic areas (East Europe, Finland, North East Asia, and Egypt), but also in US, Germany, France, and Japan.

Polyoma virus BK (BKV)

◆ Reactivation of BK virus may manifest in several different forms: asymptomatic viral replication, haemorrhagic cystitis, ureteral stricture, and viral interstitial nephritis/BK virus-associated nephropathy. This entity as a cause of kidney dysfunction is rare outside of kidney transplantation.

◆ Treatment includes the reduction of immunosuppression and specific anti-viral therapy consisting of cidofovir and leflunomide.

Other viruses

◆ Acute kidney injury complicating other viral infections is either related to multi-organ failure, rhabdomyolysis, and hepatorenal syndrome (Epstein–Barr virus, dengue fever, and typhus) or post-infectious glomerulonephritis (influenza A and hepatitis A).

◆ Epstein–Barr virus-encoded RNA 1 gene is detected in the nuclei of some tubular epithelial cells and has been speculated to be associated with the pathogenesis of chronic tubulointerstitial nephritis.

Protozoal infection

Amoebiasis

◆ The kidneys may be involved by a direct extension through the liver capsule with the development of a colonic-renal fistula, or a liver abscess draining into the kidney pelvis, or by the haematogenous route.

◆ Clinical manifestations include cystitis, haematuria, and nephritis with proteinuria and cast in urine.

Leishmaniasis (visceral)

◆ Uncommon, usually present as an atypical infection with fever, azotaemia, and proteinuria in patients with close contact with dogs.

Malaria

◆ Clinically significant kidney disorders commonly occur in infections with *Plasmodium (P.) falciparum* and *P. malariae*. Falciparum malaria causes fluid and electrolyte disorders, transient and mild glomerulonephritis, and acute kidney injury. Kidney damage is due to microcirculatory disturbance (confined to falciparum malaria) and immunological damage through the deposition of soluble IC.

◆ *P. malariae* can cause chronic glomerulopathy that may relentlessly progress to hypertension and ESRF. In contrast to acute kidney injury secondary to *P. falciparum*, anti-malarial drugs, corticosteroids, and immunosuppressive agents are not effective.

◆ Chronic malarial nephrotic syndrome seems most prevalent in adolescents, placing a heavy burden on the health services of developing countries where falciparum malaria is endemic.

◆ The pathology of the chronic form is characterized by glomerular capillary wall thickening that gradually develops to focal segmental sclerosis and finally, glomerular obsolescence and tubular atrophy. IgG, IgM, and C3 are detected in the glomerulus and one third of cases also showed malarial antigens in the glomerulus.

Schistosomiasis

◆ Glomerular disease accompanying schistosomiasis infestation occurs with *Schistosoma (S.) mansoni* and *S. japonicum*. Predominant glomerular involvement is relatively uncommon, more evident in the hepatosplenic form.

◆ Kidney disease often occurs in young subjects invariably with hepatosplenomegaly. Proteinuria (often nephrotic range) is the presenting symptom with microscopic haematuria, hypertension, and raised serum globulin in some patients.

◆ Pathologies range from mesangial thickening, focal segmental sclerosis, MCGN to crescentic glomerulonephritis. Demonstration of schistosomal antigens and elution of anti-schistosomal antibodies has been accomplished in some cases.

- The glomerulopathy is slowly progressive with little response to steroid or immunosuppressive therapy. Long-term effect of anti-schistosomal treatment is not known.

- *S. hematobium* infestation can cause chronic kidney disease through obstructive uropathy, but not via glomerulopathy.

Other parasitic infestations

- Other infestations, including toxoplasmosis, loiasis, and dioctophymiasis, have been reported to be associated with chronic kidney disease. Nephrotic syndrome has been reported and the mechanism remains unknown.

Fungal infection

- Candidiasis and aspergillosis have been reported to be associated with nephrotic syndrome. At times, this is the result of development of amyloidosis.

Chronic infective inflammation

Reflux nephropathy

Pathogenesis

- The main cause of reflux nephropathy is vesicoureteral reflux due to incompetence of the normal valvular mechanism at the vesicoureteral junction.

- Intrarenal reflux provides a mechanism whereby pathogenic organisms in the bladder urine gain access to the kidney, causing parenchymal damage and initiating scarring.

- Children with vesicoureteral reflux and urinary tract infection do not always develop reflux nephropathy. Failure to scar may depend on an insufficiency of micturating bladder pressure to cause intrarenal reflux. Children older than four years of age with vesicoureteral reflux without development of kidney scarring will not progress to reflux nephropathy.

- Vesicoureteral reflux associated with other congenital anomalies of the urinary tract is frequently complicated by kidney dysplasia.
- Late onset reflux nephropathy may occur in patients with neuropathic bladder or dysfunctional voiding.
- The grading of severity of vesicoureteral reflux, according to radiological criteria, is depicted in Table 6.4.

Clinical features

- Children with recurrent urinary tract infection.
- In later life, hypertension particularly during pregnancy or when oral contraception is started.
- Proteinuria or nephrotic syndrome if secondary focal glomerulosclerosis develops.

Pathology

- Macroscopic examination reveals coarse scars that indent the kidney surface involving cortex and medulla and directly overlie the 'clubbed' calyces shown by radiological imaging. Varying degrees of diffuse hydronephrosis with parenchymal atrophy co-exist with segmental scarring.
- Microscopically, tubulointerstitial fibrosis in scarred areas and focal glomerulosclerosis when heavy proteinuria develops.

Table 6.4 Grading system of reflux nephropathy according to the International Reflux Study Committee

Grading	Criteria
Grade I	Reflux partly up the ureter
Grade II	Reflux up to the pelvis and calyces without dilatation; normal calyceal fornices
Grade III	Same as grade II, but with mild or moderate dilatation and tortuosity of the ureter and no blunting of the fornices
Grade IV	Moderate dilatation and tortuosity of the ureter, pelvis, and calyces; complete blunting of the fornices
Grade V	Gross dilatation and tortuosity of the ureter, pelvis, and calyces; absent papillary impressions in the calyces

Treatment

- Chronic kidney disease, and even ESRF, occurs if proteinuria and hypertension persist.
- Early detection by screening for children with recurrent urinary tract infections must be stressed.
- Surgical correction of vesicoureteral reflux should be attempted in children, preferably before the age of 12.

Xanthogranulomatous pyelonephritis

- Chronic bacterial tubulointerstitial nephritis, characterized by large collections of lipid-filled foamy macrophages, granulomas, abscesses, and severe kidney parenchymal destruction. The disease is almost always unilateral.
- Predominantly affects women aged 40–60 with a history of kidney stones, recurrent urinary tract infection, obstructive uropathy, or diabetes mellitus.
- Clinical features include recurrent low-grade fever, chills, malaise, weight loss, urinary tract infection, loin pain, haematuria, cystitis, and palpable kidney mass. Occasionally, a fistula may form between the kidney and colon or skin. Urine culture almost invariably grows Gram-negative bacteria—*Proteus mirabilis* and *Escherichia (E.) coli* predominate. A lysosomal defect is suspected.
- Macroscopically, the kidney parenchyma that surrounds the dilated calyces is replaced by orange-yellow, soft inflammatory tissue, often with small abscesses. Papillae are necrotic. The inflammatory process may spread from the kidney to the retroperitoneal tissue and paracolic gutter.
- Treated by antibiotics and nephrectomy (partial or unilateral).

Malacoplakia

- Rare, chronic, bacterial tubulointerstitial nephritis, characterized by parenchymal infiltration by macrophages (von Hansemann cells) containing abundant cytoplasmic, periodic acid-Schiff-positive granules and calcified spherules known as Michaelis–Gutmann bodies. The disease is often bilateral.

- Predominantly affects middle-aged women aged 40–60 with recurrent urinary tract infections and obstruction. They are not uncommonly immunocompromised.

- Clinical features include fever, flank pain, and palpable kidneys. Bilateral disease is associated with acute kidney injury. Urine culture commonly grows *E. coli*. A lysosomal defect is suspected.

- Macroscopically, there are areas of suppuration and haemorrhage predominantly in the cortex. Extension to the medulla leads to papillary necrosis.

- Treated by antibiotics capable of intracellular penetration such as ciprofloxacin and trimethoprim, hence avoiding nephrectomy.

Megalocytic interstitial nephritis

- Cortical involvement by nodular or diffuse interstitial infiltration by large polygonal macrophages, similar to those in malacoplakia. The cellular infiltrates show fewer Michaelis–Gutmann bodies. Small, necrotizing granuloma may be seen. May represent the other end of the spectrum of malacoplakia and xanthogranulomatous pyelonephritis.

Conclusion

The relationship between infection and chronic kidney disease is an interesting subject because of the different mechanisms of glomerular and tubulointerstitial injury and heterogeneous clinicopathological patterns are operative. The aetiological role of some infective organisms is still undefined. Early identification and eradication of the infective organism are essential for preventing the development of chronic kidney disease. A continuous supply of microbial antigen and host antibody perpetuate the immunologic injury to the kidney. In the future, molecular biology techniques hold the key in further documentation of the precise nature of the infective organism in the pathogenesis of infection-related nephropathy.

Acknowledgement

Part of the work from the authors quoted in this review was supported by the L & T Charitable Fund and INDOCAFE.

References

Boonpucknavig, V., Soontornniyomkij, V., 2003. Pathology of renal diseases in the tropics. *Seminars in Nephrology*, 23(1), pp.88–106.

Bruggeman, L.A., 2007. Viral subversion mechanisms in chronic kidney disease pathogenesis. *Clinical Journal of the American Society of Nephrology*, 2(Suppl 1), S13–9.

D'Amico, G., 1998. Renal involvement in hepatitis C infection: cryoglobulinemic glomerulonephritis. *Kidney International*, 54(2), pp.650–71.

Glassock, R.J., 1991. Immune complex induced glomerular injury in viral diseases: an overview. *Kidney International*, 40(Suppl 35), S5–7.

Kimmel, P.L., Phillips, T.M., Ferreira–Centeno, A., Farkas–Szallasi, T., Abraham, A.A., Garrett, C.T., 1993. HIV-associated immune-mediated renal disease. *Kidney International*, 44(6), pp.1327–40.

Lai, A.S., Lai, K.N., 2006. Viral nephropathy. *Nature Clinical Practice Nephrology*, 2(5), pp.254–62.

Lai, K.N., Lai, F.M., 1991. Clinical features and the natural course of hepatitis B virus-related glomerulopathy in adults. *Kidney International*, 35, S40–5.

Lai, K.N., Li, P.K., Lui, S.F., Au, T.C., Tam, J.S., Tong, K.L., Lai, F.M., 1991. Membranous nephropathy related to hepatitis B virus in adults. *New England Journal of Medicine*, 324(21), pp.1457–63.

Leventhal, J.S., Ross, M.J., Lai, K.N., Tang, S.C., 2009. Glomerular disorders due to infections'. In: Lerma, V.E., Berns, J.S., Nissenson, A.R., eds. *Current diagnosis and treatment: nephrology and hypertension*. New York: McGraw–Hill, pp.296–312.

Seedat, Y.K., 2003. Glomerular disease in the tropics. *Seminars in Nephrology*, 23(1), pp.12–20.

Sitprija, V., 2003. Nephrology in Southeast Asia: fact and concept. *Kidney International*, 83, S128–30.

Chapter 7

Unique aspects of chronic kidney disease in the developing countries

Rashad Barsoum

Introduction

Chronic kidney disease (CKD) is one of the most challenging global health care problems. Underestimated for many decades, it has gradually become acknowledged as a common pathway through which many other conditions induce severe morbidity or mortality. These include diabetes, hypertension, obesity, several infections, and iatrogenic disorders.

The impact of CKD is not limited to the threat of kidney failure, but may constitute an even greater risk for cardiovascular disease (CVD) (Figure 7.1) (see Chapter 6). While this health hazard is devastating at the level of the individual, CKD has extensive socio-economic reflections on the community at large, with almost insurmountable burdens in the developing world (see Chapter 1).

Speaking of CKD in economically underprivileged nations addresses issues affecting over 80% of the world population and accounting for close to 90% of the global annual incidence of end-stage renal disease (ESRD) (Barsoum, 2002a). The particular ecological, ethnic, and socio-economic features in this vast part of the world have generated unique aspects in the epidemiology, clinical practice, and community impact, which are the focus of this chapter.

Prevalence

Since the 'Millennium' definition and classification of CKD (see Chapter 2) has been introduced by the KDOQI guidelines in 2002

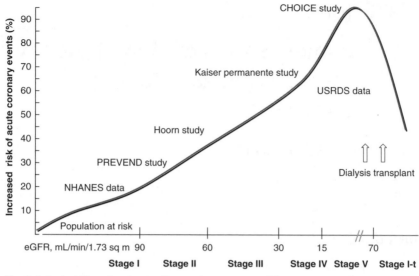

Fig. 7.1 Probability of acute cardiovascular events at different stages of CKD, assembled from reported incidence in key studies

(NKF, 2002) and the alarming data derived from NHANES III about the prevalence of CKD in the US were published (Foley, et al., 2006), epidemiological studies were conducted in almost every corner of the world, trying to identify the local CKD profile (Figure 7.2) (see Chapters 1, 4). Many of these studies were inconsistent in terms of the target population, sample size, detection thresholds, and methodology, etc. (Table 7.1), leading to widely variable figures about the prevalence, ranging from 1.39% in a rural community in India (Mani, 2005) to 31% in an apparently similar population of Tiwi aboriginals (Hoy, 2000), compared with 11% in the US (USRDS). A recent systematic review of the global figures has come up with an average of 7.2% in those older than 30 years of age and up to 35.8% in those above the age of 64. As discussed in Chapter 3, it is unclear whether age-related decline in kidney function should be considered a chronic disease or merely a physiological change.

It is noteworthy that most screening programmes have relied on single, cross-sectional testing without due consideration to the

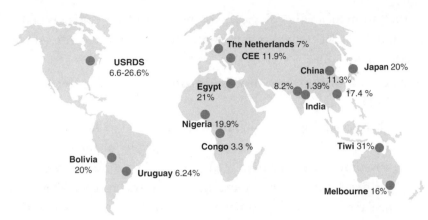

Fig. 7.2 Selected screening studies from different parts of the world showing the reported prevalence of CKD

Table 7.1 Potential bias in different screening studies for the prevalence of CKD in the developing world

Sampling bias	a. Urban or rural
	b. Hospital or field
	c. Selected groups
	d. Age/gender variations
Definition bias	a. One-time screening (CKD definition requires persistence of disease >3 months)
	b. Potential bias in the MDRD equation
	1. ? Validity in different populations
	2. ? Validity in normal range of kidney function
	3. ? validity in overweight individuals
Statistical bias	a. Sample size (power)
	b. Lack of confirmatory testing (e.g. proteinuria)
Analytical variation	a. laboratory analytical methods and reference ranges
	1. Proteinuria
	2. Serum creatinine

required confirmation of CKD by repeated testing within three months as stipulated by the KDOQI guidelines. As mentioned in Chapter 2, the true prevalence of CKD remains uncertain as the tools used so far to identify it have their limitations and have been subject of criticism.

Apart from the methodological bias, there are intrinsic reasons in the definition of CKD that may have contributed to the wide inter-study variation, including:

- Microalbuminuria vs dipstick proteinuria in the definition of CKD.
  - This logistically debatable issue (Nahas, et al., 2007) (fully discussed in Chapter 1) is certainly responsible for the significant variation in the estimation of prevalence since different studies in the developing world are inconsistent in this respect. That this bias really matters is shown by the significant difference in the NHANES III data when analyzed with transient vs persistent microalbuminuria (Bauer, et al., 2008), let alone what would the outcome be if microalbuminuria was dropped altogether as a screening test.
- Estimated glomerular filtration rate (eGFR).
  - The KDOQI CKD classification in stages 3–5 is entirely based on the eGFR, estimated by the Modified Diet in Renal Disease (MDRD) formula. While this has been validated by comparison with gold standards in low GFRs in the US, it has not in the normal ranges (Froissart, et al., 2005), particularly in other communities. Both Japanese (Imai, et al., 2007) and Chinese (Ma, et al., 2006) studies have developed their own equations by using a correction factor for reaching improved validity. The rest of the world still uses MDRD for classification without validation (Kramer, et al., 2008) (the limitations of this equation and estimated GFR is fully discussed in Chapter 2).
- Serum creatinine.
  - Since most studies are based on single readings of serum creatinine for the estimation of GRF, any methodological errors or transient changes would significantly modify the outcome. It is noteworthy that the measurement of serum creatinine is subject to considerable variations, depending on the analytical method which varies in different locations. Serum creatinine may also vary, even in the same individual, depending on age,

nutritional and hydration status, muscular exercise, and other factors which are particularly prominent in the developing world.

Risk factors

The risk factors for CKD are quite different in the developing world from those in the industrialized nations (Table 7.2). While diabetes and hypertension are leading in the latter, glomerulonephritis and interstitial nephritis due to obstruction, infection, or drug abuse are more relevant in the developing world (Barsoum, 2002b). The relative significance of these factors is variable according to ethnic variations, regional bioecology, environmental pollution, and socio-economic conditions that directly reflect on primary health care.

Ethnicity

There is evidence that blacks and indigenous populations (Nicholas, et al., 2005) in different parts of the world are more vulnerable to CKD, which rapidly progresses to ESRD, and is responsible for a significantly increased incidence of cardiovascular complications. There are several explanations for these observations, including genetic factors, low birthweight, lower socio-economic standards, and limited availability of primary health care to the majority (Norris & Nissenson, 2008).

Table 7.2 Major risk factors for CKD in the developing world

Typical global factors with escalating impact in the developing world	a. Hypertension b. Diabetes (growing profile) c. Smoking d. Obesity

Specific factors mostly prevalent in the developing world	a. Ethnic predisposition
	b. Infections
	  1. Viral (e.g. HIV, HCV, HBV, etc.)
	  2. Bacterial (e.g. streptococcal, enteric, etc.)
	  3. Parasitic (schistosomiasis, malaria, onchocerciasis, etc.)
	c. Environmental pollution (?)
	d. Compromised primary health care

Bioecology

Infection is responsible for a considerable proportion of CKD in endemic areas (Figure 7.3). A striking example is HIV, which currently affects up to 20% of the adult population and 17–38% of women attending antenatal care clinics in sub-Saharan Africa (Katz, 2005). Nephropathy is reported in 3–10% of HIV-infected individuals, accounting for 6–38% (Emem, et al., 2008; Naicker, et al., 2006) of the overall incidence of CKD. HIV is largely replaced by hepatitis C virus (HCV) at the northern end of the same continent, with a prevalence of 20% in Egypt, an expected incidence of glomerular lesions in over 50% of cases (Arase, et al., 1998), and actually accounting for about 40% of mesangiocapillary (membranoproliferative) glomerulonephritis in the same country (Sabry, et al., 2005). This sharp contrast in the prevalence and renal pathogenicity of two common viral infections is yet one of the striking examples of the effect of bioecology on CKD. Similarly variable impact of other infections is observed in different parts of the developing world (Barsoum & Sitprija, 2007) (Figure 7.3).

Regional bioecology is not constant. Changes in weather conditions, geological modification by dams and artificial lakes, human behaviour, and disease control programmes have often resulted in, and will continue to impose, significant modifications in the CKD risk profile in the

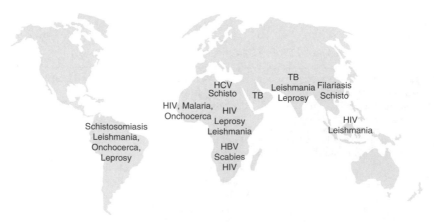

Fig. 7.3 Epidemiologically significant infections responsible for CKD in different parts of the developing world

developing world. For example, schistosomiasis that was once held responsible for one third of CKD in Egypt, has now regressed to less than 8% (Egyptian Society of Nephrology, 2006), on its way to vanish under the pressure of effective control programmes. Unfortunately, this profile is not consistent in other parts of the world, as in China where man-made ecological changes are expected to increase the prevalence of schistosomiasis following an initial decline due to mass treatment programmes (World Health Organization, 2004). Similar models apply to other highly prevalent diseases in the developing world as malaria, tuberculosis, filariasis, and other infections (see Chapter 5).

Environmental pollution

The majority of big cities in the developing world have a high level of air pollution while the villages often suffer significant water pollution. Many environmental contaminants have been shown in experimental models to cause chronic interstitial disease. It is difficult to extrapolate these models to humans owing to differences in body size, relevant metabolic pathways, duration of exposure, and other factors (Barsoum & Sitprija, 2007). However, the high incidence of unexplained chronic interstitial disease in many series from the developing world keeps this question open for further studies.

Socio-economic conditions

The supervening standards of health care have a direct impact on the prevalence of CKD, which reflects the ability of early detection and management of underlying disorders. There are several components in primary health care, including the number and capacity of professionals, facilities, administrative competence, and budgets. Shortage in all of these aspects is a dominant feature in most developing world countries. A look into the health budgets (World Bank, 2002) of some of these countries (Figure 7.4) highlights such discrepancies.

It is even more alarming that the prevailing poor socio-economic standards will add long-term risk factors in the near future. Low birthweights, malnutrition, increasing incidence of hypertension (Ibrahim, et al., 1995), diabetes (Wild, et al., 2004), obesity and the metabolic

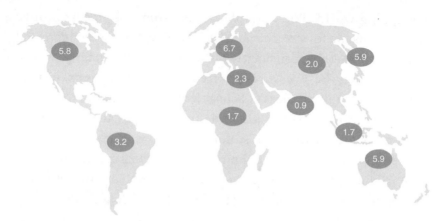

Fig. 7.4 Percentage of GDP allotted to public sector health care in different countries

syndrome, (Hossain, et al., 2007) and the escalating prevalence of smoking among the young (Abdullah, et al., 2004) are smouldering factors that anticipate a dramatic increase in the prevalence of CKD in the coming few decades.

Diagnosis

The vast majority of CKD patients are referred to the nephrologist while already in stage 5. This reflects the dearth of awareness among primary health care providers who fail to detect early CKD as well as among specialists who delay the referral of high-risk patients such as those with diabetes or hypertension, deliberately or unknowingly. This raises the question about the optimal timing for referring patients with known CKD. While KDOQI guidelines suggest this to occur at the onset of stage 3, it may not be possible in developing countries where nephrologists are too few and the patients too many.

It follows that any national plan should involve the primary health care providers and relevant specialists in the process of early diagnosis and management. This should entail raising awareness about CKD, particularly among high-risk patients, developing comprehensive plans for their follow-up, implementing standard treatment strategies, and setting thresholds for referral to a nephrologist.

Table 7.3 Conditions most frequently associated with undiagnosed CKD in the developing world

Underlying disease	Diabetes
	Hypertension
	Excessive obesity
	Endemic infection
Mistaken manifestations of CKD	Anaemia
	Gastrointestinal disorders
	Premature CVD
	Unexplained osteoporosis

Awareness is the key issue (Table 7.3). Non-nephrologists should routinely assess their patients for CKD if: they have one of the common diseases which are known to lead to CKD such as diabetes, hypertension or if they are obese; they have one of the local endemic diseases known to be associated with CKD such as HIV, HCV, schistosomiasis, malaria, etc.; or they have a clinical manifestation of CKD that may be mistakenly attributed to another common aetiology in a particular community such as anaemia, osteopaenia, recurrent vomiting, or abdominal complaints, etc. Exclusion of CKD in these patients does not need special skills or sophisticated equipment, just awareness. Many protocols have been put forward for early diagnosis, all of which share the simplicity of the initial screening being limited to the examination of midstream urine, measurement of serum creatinine with a calculation of the eGFR, and performing a simple, ultrasonic imaging (International Society of Nephrology, 2004; NKF, 2002].

It is also important to realize that, while the non-nephrologist takes over the task of management in early CKD, comorbid conditions often confound its clinical features and natural history. These include malnutrition, chronic infections, drug abuse, and other organ disorders such as liver, heart, or lung disease. A clear account of these disorders must constitute an integral part of the diagnosis.

A follow-up plan for the progression of CKD must be developed, depending upon the nature of the disease, its rate of progression, and confounding factors. The threshold for referral to nephrology should be agreed upon at a national level, depending on the availability of facilities and personnel. Generally, as mentioned earlier, stage 3 is the optimal threshold since it requires a certain experience in dealing with the metabolic and haemodynamic consequences of impaired renal function. However, many studies have shown that the rate of progression of CKD and the associated risk of cardiovascular disease are different in early as opposed to late stage 3, the transition being 45mL/min. For this reason, stage III may be conveniently divided into 3a (45–59mL/min) and 3b (30–44mL/min). With some additional training, the primary care physician should be able to manage stage 3a patients along the same lines for stages 1 and 2.

Treatment options

The general management plan for early CKD, recommended by most clinical practice guidelines (CPGs), is largely based on published randomized control trials (RCTs) (Manley, 2007). It is noteworthy that while these recommendations are strongly evidence-based in patients with diabetic CKD (Brenner, et al., 2001; Lewis, et al., 2001), their extrapolation to non-diabetic populations is often circumstantial. It is interesting that RCTs addressing many of these recommendations in non-diabetic CKD populations have come up with inconclusive results (Kaisar, et al., 2008), particularly in the absence of proteinuria (<1g/24h). Nevertheless, long-term observational studies suggest that adequate blood pressure control (Sarnak, et al., 2005) and the use of renin-angiotensin-aldosterone system (RAAS) blockade (Appel, et al., 2008; Balamuthusamy, et al., 2008) in such patients may reduce cardiovascular mortality, yet with questionable effect on the pooled rate of CKD progression. On the other hand, there is fairly strong evidence that angiotensin-converting enzyme inhibitors (ACEis) slow the progression of CKD in IgA nephropathy and primary FSGS, HIV nephropathy (Burns, et al., 1997), and less impressively, in other forms of chronic glomerulonephritis. ACEis ameliorate interstitial fibrosis in rats with partial unilateral ureteric obstruction (Koo, et al., 2003), a model that is very similar to clinical disease associated with schistosomiasis or tuberculosis. However, clinical correlates are lacking.

Interventional studies addressing other risk factors generally lack hard end points despite showing improvement of surrogate metabolic markers. Having mentioned that and until hard evidence is available, it should be safe to adopt the KEEP recommendations in the developing world, with due consideration to the supervening confounding factors.

The KEEP study (Manley, 2007) concluded that the three main categories of intervention must be applied to all CKD patients:, namely changes in lifestyle, achievement of well-defined numerical targets, and specific intervention for cardiovascular complications (Table 7.4).

Table 7.4 Principal targets in the management of CKD

Management of underlying disease	
Management of reversible confounding factors	
Lifestyle modification	
Diet	See Table 7.4
Weight control	As near ideal as possible
Exercise	20min/day, 30min alternate days
Cessation of smoking	
Meeting numerical targets	
Blood pressure	<130/80 non-diabetic; <120/70 diabetic
HbA1c	<7.0%
Cholesterol	Total <200mg/dL, LDL <100mg/dL, HDL >45mg/dL
Triglycerides	<500mg/dL
Haemoglobin	11–12g/dL
Ferritin	200mg/dL
Ca	8.4–9.5mg/dL
Pi	2.7–4.6mg/dL; Ca x P <55
PTH	Intact molecule 35–70 in stage 3, 70–110 in stage 4
Bicarbonate	22–24mmol/L
Pharmacological agents (see text for debates)	
Agents for control of diabetes, hypertension, etc.	Diabetic kidney disease, proteinuria >1g/24h
RAAS inhibitors	
Statins	

Table 7.5 Dietary approaches to Stop Hypertension (DASH) diet

	Stages I, II	Stages III, IV
Protein g/kg/d (% of Cal)	1.4 (18)	0.6–0.8 (10)
Total fat (% of Cal)	<30	
Saturated fat (% of Cal)	<10	
Cholesterol (mg/d)	<200	
Carbohydrate (% of Cal)	50–60	
Phosphorus (g/d)	1.7	0.8–1.0
Potassium (g/d)	>4	2–4
Sodium (g/d)	<2.4	

- ◆ Lifestyle modification.
  - • The DASH-Sodium diet (Phillips, et al., 1999) has been strongly recommended in the KDOQI guidelines (NKF, 2002). This is basically a low fat, protein-adjusted diet, rich in fruits and vegetables with severe salt restriction (Table 7.5). It is important to avoid undue protein-calorie malnutrition in those patients, which is a common mistake in the developing world, leading to serious long-term consequences that may extend to later stages of CKD. Weight control can be achieved by a gradual caloric restriction. While the achievement of the ideal body weight is an ultimate goal, this may not be possible in many patients. A few pounds less in body weight is an acceptable alternative since it confers considerable cardiovascular protection. Gentle exercise for 20 minutes daily or 30 minutes on alternate days is recommended. Walking, jogging, swimming, or gardening are generally preferred and well tolerated by most patients. Smoking cessation is of vital importance in the interest of both CKD progression and cardiovascular complications; no compromise should be accepted.
- ◆ Meeting numerical targets.
  - • Most CPGs have set numerical targets in the control of blood pressure, haemoglobin concentration, plasma lipids, calcium,

phosphate, and parathyroid hormone (PTH) levels. Most of these are achievable by the appropriate use of medications (see Chapter 8). Guidelines also agree that regardless of the numerical targets, RAAS blockade must be attempted in all patients with diabetic and/or proteinuric CKD, unless contraindicated, because of hyperkalaemia, acidosis, bilateral renal artery stenosis, or drug side effects. RAAS inhibitors should be used with caution in elderly patients who often have diffuse atherosclerotic disease with increased risk of renal vascular disease, which predisposes to an acute deterioration of kidney function upon treatment with these agents. Both ACEis and angiotensin receptor I blockers (ARBs) may be used alone or in combination. There is some, though inconclusive, evidence that their effects be additive in reducing proteinuria.

- ◆ Specific intervention for cardiovascular complications.
  - • Patients with symptoms or signs suggestive of CVD must be assessed by their respective specialists. According to conclusions from the KEEP study, aspirin prophylaxis must be used in patients with particularly high cardiovascular risk and beta-adrenergic blockers in those who actually had previous myocardial infarctions. It has also been argued that in view of the fact that patients with advanced CKD are at a high CVD risk, they ought to be treated with statins (see Chapter 5). However, evidence to support such contention is still lacking and the cost-effectiveness of such approach has not been validated.

Treatment of the cause

Several case-control studies suggest that early treatment of the cause of CKD may lead to regression or stabilization for many decades. This has been documented in many forms of active glomerulonephritis, including systemic lupus erythematosus (SLE), vasculitis, obstructive disease, iatrogenic nephropathies, and early infection-related glomerulopathies such as those associated with schistosomiasis, HCV, HBV, HIV, and others. Despite the lack of hard evidence, it makes good sense to treat an active disease associated with CKD, even if the course of the latter is not altered by such treatment.

Management of Stages III-b and IV

The progression of CKD towards end-stage is the rule in patients reaching this level of compromised function, unless they expire, as most do, from another cause, often CVD. Although a reversal of ongoing pathology may still be possible, the risk of aggressive treatment must be weighed against the expected benefit. The general recommendations apply with even more stringent adherence to blood pressure control, haemoglobin levels, and biochemical targets. While the effect on progression of dietary protein targets lower that those recommended in the K/DOQI-modified DASH diet (NKF, 2002) has not been confirmed (Levey, et al., 2006), they may confer symptomatic benefit by reducing several metabolic derangements in CKD (Cianciaruso, et al., 2008). On the basis of the latter study, the net protein intake may be reduced to 0.55g/kg/day, not any further, in order to avoid malnutrition. Unless there is a clear contraindication such as hyperkalaemia or acidosis, RAAS inhibitors should be continued despite the deteriorating function, within the limits of 20–30% decline of eGFR in three months compared to the pre-treatment level.

Management of Stage V

Renal replacement therapy (RRT) should be considered in each patient crossing the stage 5 cut-off line. Unfortunately, many countries in the developing world can afford providing this treatment only to a few. In response to such shortage, some countries have developed rationing models for prioritization (Barsoum, et al., 1974), others yield under the pressure of political, social or financial power (Farid, et al., 1993), and still others stay helpless, restricting RRT to acute kidney injury.

All modalities of RRT are offered to a variable extent in different parts of the developing world (Barsoum, 2002b) (Figure 7.5). Overall, this is largely dependent on prevailing socio-economic standards (Barsoum, 2006). Haemodialysis is, by far, the most prevalent modality, though chronic ambulatory peritoneal dialysis (CAPD) is offered preferentially in a few countries such as South Africa, Mexico, and Hong Kong (Barsoum, 2002b). Transplantation is offered only in the better-off countries where the facilities and personnel are available. Deceased donor

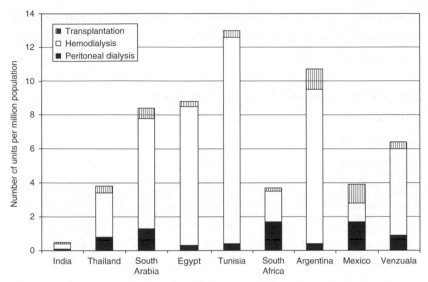

Fig. 7.5 Prevalence of units providing different modalities of RRT in selected developing world countries

programmes are available in a few countries where legislation is established, with adequate public awareness and blessing by the religious leaders. In quite a few, only living donors are available, being either related or unrelated. The latter have created a lot of negative social impact, encouraged transplant commercialism, tourism, and organ trafficking (Barsoum, 2008). A lot of international effort is currently underway to limit this shameful practice. Of many announcements and position statements published over the past decade, the strongest is the 2008 Istanbul Declaration (2008).

The outcomes of RRT in the developing world are generally less favourable than those reported in the industrialized world (Barsoum, 2004), due to late patient referral, shortage of equipment, medications and trained personnel, and the developing world confounding factors described earlier.

Unfortunately, the financial burden of ESRD management on developing countries has imposed considerable compromises in the availability and quality of services, and created plenty of friction among the funding bodies, physicians, and patient organizations. There are many models for involving non-governmental organizations, insurance companies, and philanthropic groups in lifting part of the burden off the States' shoulders with varying levels of success (Barsoum, 2002b).

The socio-economic impact of prevention programmes

Following the fever of detection of CKD in different parts of the developing world, millions of patients at risk or already in different stages of CKD were identified. These impose a clear moral commitment on the community to provide preventive measures, including the treatment of the primary disease, reducing risk factors, and providing standard treatments aiming at well-defined targets. This has actually been implemented in different parts of the developing world, with impressive models in Bolivia (Plata, et al., 1998) and India (Mani, 2005).

While the implementation of adequate treatment should reduce cardiovascular and all-cause mortality, it is uncertain if it will reduce the incidence of RRT, decades ahead. Indeed, there is concern that the latter may actually increase as patients live long enough after eliminating non-renal causes of death, including CVD. Accordingly, the dream of reducing the cost of RRT by adequate prevention may turn to become a nightmare to the health authorities that will have to provide treatment to millions of asymptomatic patients in addition to a possibly increased burden of RRT. This has raised the question whether the medical profession has gone too far by equating risk with disease, thereby unnecessarily treating healthy individuals. After all, the available funds will not change that much in the near future and the implementation of mass treatment programmes in stages 1 and 2 may have negative reflections on other areas of medical care, including ESRD itself.

Therefore, it seems logical to recommend limiting the screening for CKD to high-risk subjects. Missing low-risk subjects in early stages of CKD would not have a significant health impact since the majority of those subjects may not progress to later stages, and their risk of developing CVD is low.

References

Abdullah, A.S., Husten, C.G., 2004. Promotion of smoking cessation in developing countries: a framework for urgent public health interventions. *Thorax*, 59(7), pp.623–30.

Appel, L.J., Wright, J.T. Jr, Greene, T., Kusek, J.W., Lewis, J.B., Wang, X., Lipkowitz, M.S., Norris, K.C., Bakris, G.L., Rahman, M., Contreras, G., Rostand, S.G., Kopple, J.D., Gabbai, F.B., Schulman, G.I., Gassman, J.J., Charleston, J., Adogoa, L.Y.; African American Study of Kidney Disease and Hypertension Collaborative Research Group, 2008. Long-term effects of renin-angiotensin system-blocking therapy and a low blood pressure goal on progression of hypertensive chronic kidney disease in African Americans. *Archives of Internal Medicine*, 168(8), pp.832–9.

Arase, Y., Ikeda, K., Murashima, N., Chayama, K., Tsubota, A., Koida, I., Suzuki, Y., Saitoh, S., Kobayashi, M., Kobayashi, M., Kobayashi, M., Kumuda, H., 1998. Glomerulonephritis in autopsy cases with hepatitis C virus infection. *Internal Medicine*, 37(10), pp.836–40.

Arogundade, F.A., Barsoum, R.S., 2008. CKD prevention in Sub-Saharan Africa: a call for governmental, nongovernmental, and community support. *American Journal of Kidney Diseases*, 51(3), pp.515–23.

Balamuthusamy, S., Srinivasan, L., Verma, M., Adigopula, S., Jalandhara, N., Hathiwala, S., Smith, E., 2008. Renin angiotensin system blockade and cardiovascular outcomes in patients with chronic kidney disease and proteinuria: a meta-analysis. *American Heart Journal*, 155(5), pp.791–805.

Barsoum, R.S., Rihan, Z.E., Ibrahim, A.S., Lebstein, A., 1974. Long-term intermittent haemodialysis in Egypt. *Bulletin of the World Health Organization*, 51(6), pp.647–54.

Barsoum, R.S., 2002a. End-stage renal disease in the developing world (editorial). *Artificial Organs*, 26(9), pp.735–6

Barsoum, R.S., 2002b. Overview: end-stage renal disease in the developing world. *Artificial Organs*, 26(9), pp.737–46.

Barsoum, R.S., 2004. Dialysis in the developing world. In: Horl, W.H., Koch, K., Lindsay, R., Ronco, C., Winchester, J., eds. *Replacement of renal function by dialysis*. 5th ed. New York/Heidelberg: Springer, 58, pp.1487–95.

Barsoum, R.S., 2006. Chronic kidney disease in the developing world. *New England Journal of Medicine*, 354(10), pp.997–9.

Barsoum, R., Sitprija, V., 2007. Tropical nephrology. In: Schrier, R.W., ed. *Diseases of the kidney and urinary tract*. 3rd ed. Philadelphia: Lippincott Williams & Wilkins, 78, pp.2013–55.

Barsoum, R.S., 2008. Trends in unrelated-donor kidney transplantation in the developing world. *Pediatric Nephrology*, 23(11), pp.1925–9.

Bauer, C., Melamed, M.L., Hostetter, T.H., 2008. Staging of chronic kidney disease: time for a course correction. *Journal of the American Society of Nephrology*, 19(5), pp.844–6.

Brenner, B.M., Cooper, M.E., de Zeeuw D., Keane, W.F., Mitch, W.E., Parving, H.H., Remuzzi, G., Snapinn, S.M., Zhang, A., Shahinfar, S.; RENAAL Study Investigators, 2001. Effects of losartan on renal and cardiovascular outcomes in patients with type 2 diabetes and nephropathy. *New England Journal of Medicine*, 345(12), pp.861–9.

Burns, G.C., Paul, S.K., Toth, I.R., Sivak, S.L., 1997. Effect of angiotensin-converting enzyme inhibition in HIV-associated nephropathy. *Journal of the American Society of Nephrology*, 8(7), pp.1140–6.

Chadban, S.J., Briganti, E.M., Kerr, P.G., Dunstan, D.W., Welborn, T.A., Zimmet, P.Z., Atkins, R.C., 2003. Prevalence of kidney damage in Australian adults: The AusDiab kidney study. *Journal of the American Society of Nephrology*, 14(7 Suppl 2), S131–8.

Cianciaruso, B., Pota, A., Pisani, A., Torraca, S., Annecchini, R., Lombardi, P., Capuano, A., Nazzaro, P., Bellizzi, V., Sabbatini, M., 2008. Metabolic effects of two low protein diets in chronic kidney disease stage 4-5—a randomized controlled trial. *Nephrology Dialysis Transplantation*, 23(2), pp.636–44.

Egyptian Society of Nephrology, 2006. *Annual report 2006*. [Online] Available at: http://www.esnonline.net/ [Accessed 15 July 2008].

Emem, C.P., Arogundade, F., Sanusi, A., Adelusola, K., Wokoma, F., Akinsola, A., 2008. Renal disease in HIV-seropositive patients in Nigeria: an assessment of prevalence, clinical features and risk factors. Nephrology *Dialysis Transplantation*, 23(2), pp.741–6.

Farid, M.T., Torky, A.H., Barsoum, R.S., 1993. Psychological profiles in related and unrelated live kidney donors. *Proceedings of the 2nd International Congress of Geographical Nephrology*. Hurghada, Egypt [February 1993].

Foley, R., Wang, C., Ishani, A., Collins, A., Murray, A., 2007. Kidney function & sarcopenia in the United States general population: the NHANES III Study. *American Journal of Nephrology*, 27(3), pp.279–86.

Froissart, M., Rossert, J., Jacquot, C., Paillard, M., Houillier, P., 2005. Predictive performance of the modification of diet in renal disease and Cockcroft-Gault equations for estimating renal function. *Journal of the American Society of Nephrology*, 16(3), pp.763–73.

Go, A.S., Chertow, G.M., Fan, D., McCullough, C.E., Hsu, C.Y., 2004. Chronic kidney disease and the risks of death, cardiovascular events, and hospitalization. *New England Journal of Medicine*, 351(13), pp.1296–305.

Gouda, Z.E., Elattar, A., Elbaz, Z., 2007. Egypt information, prevention and treatment of chronic kidney diseases (EGYPT-CKD) Project. World Congress of Nephrology, Rio De Janeiro, Brazil, 21–25 April 2007. Abstract T-PO-1225.

Henry, R.M., Kostense, P.J., Bos, G., Dekker, J.M., Nijpels, G., Heine, R.J., Bouter, L.M., Stehouwer, C.D., 2002. Mild renal insufficiency is associated with increased cardiovascular mortality: the Hoorn Study. *Kidney International*, 62(4), pp.1402–7.

Hillege, H.L., Fidler, V., Diercks, G.F., van Gilst, W.H., de Zeeuw, D., van Veldhuisen, D.J., Gans, R.O., Janssen, W.M., Grobbee, D.E., de Jong, P.E.; Prevention of Renal and Vascular End-Stage Disease (PREVEND) Study Group, 2002. Urinary albumin excretion predicts cardiovascular and non-cardiovascular mortality in general population. *Circulation*, 106(14), pp.1777–82.

Hossain, P., Kawar, B., El Nahas, M., 2007. Obesity and diabetes in the developing world—a growing challenge. *New England Journal of Medicine*, 356(3), pp.213–5.

Hoy, W., 2000. Renal disease in Australian Aborigines. *Nephrology Dialysis Transplantation*, 15(9), pp.1293–7.

Ibrahim, M.M., Rizk, H., Appel, L.J., el Aroussy, W., Helmy, S., Sharaf, Y., Ashour, Z., Kandil, H., Roccella, E., Whelton, P.K., 1995. Hypertension prevalence, awareness, treatment, and control in Egypt. Results from the Egyptian National Hypertension Project (NHP). *Hypertension*, 26(6), pp.886–90.

Imai, E., Horio, M., Nitta, K., Yamagata, K., Iseki, K., Hara, S., Ura, N., Kiyohara, Y., Hirakata, H., Watanabe, T., Moriyama, T., Ando, Y., Inaguma, D., Narita, I., Iso, H., Wakai, K., Yasuda, Y., Tsukamoto, Y., Ito, S., Makino, H., Hishida, A., Matsuo, S., 2007. Estimation of glomerular filtration rate by the MDRD study equation modified for Japanese patients with chronic kidney disease. *Clinical and Experimental Nephrology*, 11(1), pp.41–50.

International Society of Nephrology, 2004. ISN programme for detection and management of chronic kidney disease, hypertension, diabetes, and cardiovascular disease in developing countries (KHDC). [Online] Available at: http://www.nature.com/isn/education/guidelines/isn/pdf/ed_051027_2x1.pdf [Accessed 15 June 2008].

International Summit on Transplant Tourism and Organ Trafficking, 2008. The Declaration of Istanbul on organ trafficking and transplant tourism. *Kidney International*, 74(7), pp.854–9.

Iseki, K., 2008. Chronic kidney disease in Japan. *Internal Medicine*, 47(8), pp.681–9.

Jones, C.A., McQuillan, G.M., Kusek, J.W., Eberhardt, M.S., Herman, W.H., Coresh, J., Salive, M., Jones, C.P., Agodoa, L.Y., 1998. Serum creatinine levels in the US population: third National Health and Nutrition Examination Survey. *American Journal of Kidney Diseases*, 32(6), pp.992–9.

Kaisar, M.O., Isbel, N.M., Johnson, D.W., 2008. Recent clinical trials of pharmacologic cardiovascular interventions in patients with chronic kidney disease. *Reviews on Recent Clinical Trials*, 3(2), pp.79–88.

Katz, I., 2005. Kidney and kidney related chronic diseases in South Africa and chronic disease intervention program experiences. *Advances in Chronic Kidney Disease*, 121(1), pp.14–21.

Koo, J.W., Kim, Y., Rozen, S., Mauer, M., 2003. Enalapril accelerates remodeling of the renal interstitium after release of unilateral ureteral obstruction in rats. *Journal of Nephrology*, 16(2), pp.203–9.

Kramer, H., Palmas, W., Kestenbaum, B., Cushman, M., Allison, M., Astor, B., Shlipak, M., 2008. Chronic kidney disease prevalence estimates among racial/ethnic groups: the multi-ethnic study of atherosclerosis. *Clinical Journal of the American Society of Nephrology*, 3(5), pp.1391–7.

Krzesinski, J.M., Sumaili, K.E., Cohen, E., 2007. How to tackle the avalanche of chronic kidney disease in sub-Saharan Africa: the situation in the Democratic Republic of Congo as an example. *Nephrology Dialysis Transplantation*, 22(2), pp.332–5.

Levey, A.S., Greene, T., Sarnak, M.J., Wang, X., Beck, G.J., Kusek, J.W., Collins, A.J., Kopple, J.D., 2006. Effect of dietary protein restriction on the progression of kidney disease: long-term follow-up of the Modification of Diet in Renal Disease (MDRD) Study. *American Journal of Kidney Diseases*, 48(6), pp.879–88.

Lewis, E.J., Hunsicker, L.G., Clarke, W.R., Berl, T., Pohl, M.A., Lewis, J.B., Ritz, E., Atkins, R.C., Rohde, R., Raz, I.; Collaborative Study Group, 2001. Renoprotective effect of the angiotensin-receptor antagonist irbesartan in patients with nephropathy due to type 2 diabetes. *New England Journal of Medicine*, 345(12), pp.851–60.

Longenecker, J.C., Coresh, J., Powe, N.R., Levey, A.S., Fink, N.E., Martin, A., Klag, M.J., 2002. Traditional cardiovascular disease risk factors in dialysis patients compared with the general population: the CHOICE Study. *Journal of the American Society of Nephrology*, 13(7), pp.1918–27.

Ma, Y.C., Zuo, L., Chen, J.H., Luo, Q., Yu, X.Q., Li, Y., Xu, J.S., Huang, S.M., Wang, L.N., Huang, W., Wang, M., Xu, G.B.,Wang, H.Y., 2006. Modified glomerular filtration rate estimating equation for Chinese patients with chronic kidney disease. *Journal of the American Society of Nephrology*, 17(10), pp.2937–44.

Mani, M.K., 2005. Experience with a program for prevention of chronic renal failure in India. *Kidney International Suppl*, (94), S75–8.

Manley, H.J., 2007. Disease progression and the application of evidence-based treatment guidelines diagnose it early: a case for screening and appropriate management. *Journal of Managed Care Pharmacy*, 13(9 Suppl D), S6–12.

Nahas, A.M., Kawar, B., El-Kossi, M., 2007. Chronic kidney disease–Into the 21st century. European Renal Disease 2007; 1(1), pp.10–12.

Naicker, S., Han, T.M., Fabian, J., 2006. HIV/AIDS–dominant player in chronic kidney disease. *Ethnicity and Disease*, 16(2 Suppl 2), S2-56–60.

National Kidney Foundation, 2002. KDOQI clinical practice guidelines for chronic kidney disease: evaluation, classification, and stratification. *American Journal of Kidney Diseases*, 39(2 Suppl 1), S1–266.

Nicholas, S.B., Tareen, N., Zadshir, A., Martins, D., Pan, D., Norris, K.C., 2005. Management of early chronic kidney disease in indigenous populations and ethnic minorities. *Kidney International Suppl*, (97), S78–81.

Norris, K., Nissenson, A., 2008. Racial disparities in chronic kidney disease: tragedy, opportunity, or both? *Clinical Journal of the American Society of Nephrology*, 3(2), pp.314–6.

Phillips, K.M., Stewart, K.K., Karanja, N.M., Windhauser, M.M., Champagne, C.M., Swain, J.F., Lin, P.H., Evans, M.A., 1999. Validation of diet composition for the Dietary Approaches to Stop Hypertension trial. DASH Collaborative Research Group. *Journal of the American Dietetic Association*, 99(8 Suppl), S60–8.

Plata, R., Silva, C., Yahuita, J., Perez, L., Schieppati, A., Remuzzi, G., 1998. The first clinical and epidemiological programme on renal disease in Bolivia: a model for prevention and early diagnosis of renal diseases in the developing countries. *Nephrology Dialysis Transplantation*, 13(12), pp.3034–6.

Rutkowski, B., Król, E., 2008. Epidemiology of Chronic Kidney Disease in Central and Eastern Europe. *Blood Purification*, 26(4), pp.381–5.

Sabry, A., El-Agroudy, A., Sheashaa, H., El-Husseini, A., Taha, N.M., Elbaz, M., El-Shahat, F., Sobh, M., 2005. Histological characterization of HCV-associated glomerulopathy in Egyptian patients. *International Urology and Nephrology*, 37(2), pp.355–61.

Sarnak, M.J., Greene, T., Wang, X., Beck, G., Kusek, J.W., Collins, A.J., Levey, A.S., 2005. The effect of a lower target blood pressure on the progression of kidney disease: long-term follow-up of the modification of diet in renal disease study. *Annals in Internal Medicine*, 142(5), pp.342–51.

Singh, N.P., Ajita, G., Ingle, G.K., Beniwal, P., 2007. Prevalence of Chronic Kidney Disease (CKD) and its associated risk factors in and around Delhi. World Congress of Nephrology, Rio De Janeiro, Brazil, 21–25 April 2007 [Abstract T-PO-1260].

Sola, L., Stoll, M., Bankoff, L., Mariani, A., Noboa, O., Sehabiagne, C., Pastorino, A., Orihuela, L., De Souza, N., Boghossian, S., Abadie, S. 2007. High prevalence of cardiovascular and kidney disease risk factors in relatives of dialysis patients. World Congress of Nephrology, Rio De Janeiro, Brazil, 21–25 April 2007 [Abstract T-PO-1310].

United States Renal Data System (USRDS), 2003. *Kidney Transplant Follow-ups-UNOS*. [Online] Available at: http://www. usrds.org/default.asp [Accessed 14 Jan 2005].

Wei, H., Horng, S., Shiu, R., Wu, S., Tu, Y., Hsiao, M., Chang, P., Hwang, S. 2007. Risk Factors Associated with Self-Reported Kidney Diseases in Taiwan- Study from the 2005 National Health Survey. World Congress of Nephrology, Rio De Janeiro, Brazil, 21–25 April 2007 [Abstract T-PO-1145].

Wild, S., Roglic, G., Green, A., Sicree, R., King, H., 2004. Global prevalence of diabetes: estimates for the year 2000 and projections for 2030. *Diabetes Care*, 27(5), pp.1047–53.

World Bank, 2002. *Country reports 2002*. [Online] Available at: http://web.worldbank. org [Accessed 15 July 2008].

World Health Organization, 2004. *Schistosomiasis*. [Online] Available at: http://www. who.int/tdr/svc/diseases/schistosomiasis [Accessed 15 July 2008].

Zhang, L., Zuo, L., Xu, G., Wang, F., Wang, M., Wang, S., Lv, J., Liu, J., Wang, H., 2007. Community-based screening for chronic kidney disease among populations older than 40 years in Beijing. *Nephrology Dialysis Transplantation*, 22(4), pp.1093–9.

Chapter 8

Management of chronic kidney disease: controlling hypertension and reducing proteinuria

Aimun Ahmed, Fairol H. Ibrahim, and
Meguid El Nahas

Introduction

Over the last decade, increased awareness of chronic kidney disease
(CKD) has stemmed from a new classification introduced in 2002 by
the National Kidney Foundation/Kidney Disease Outcomes Quality
Initiative (KDOQI) based on levels of glomerular filtration rate (GFR)
and the presence of evidence of kidney damage such as albuminuria or
haematuria (KDOQI, 2002).

The CKD classification with the subsequent increased interest in the
detection of CKD has prompted a number of cohort studies aimed at
determining factors in communities affecting the incidence of CKD
(see Chapter 3). Of the risk factors associated with the development
and progression of CKD, systemic hypertension has the mostpromi-
nent and causal link. Along with systemic hypertension, proteinuria has
also been shown to be a predictor of progressive CKD. In addition, the
prevention and reduction of hypertension and proteinuria are, respectively, considered the cornerstones of the prevention and management
of CKD.

Hypertension and the risk of development of CKD

A number of community-based studies have identified modifiable
markers/factors associated with increased risk of developing CKD (see
Chapter 3).

Table 8.1 KDOQI CKD classification (KDOQI, 2002)

Stage	Description	GFR (mL/min/1.73m^2)
1	Kidney damage with normal or increased GFR	≥90
2	Kidney damage with mildly decreased GFR	60–89
3	Moderately decreased GFR	30–59
4	Severely decreased GFR	15–29
5	Kidney failure	<15 (or dialysis)

NB. The National Institute of Health and Clinical Excellence (NICE) CKD guideline issued in 2008 recommended to subdivide stage 3 into stage 3a (GFR 59–45mL/min/1.73m^2) and 3b (GFR 44–30mL/min/1.73m^2), and to add the suffix 'p' to the stage in proteinuric patients (Crowe, et al., 2008).

Foremost among CKD risk factors in communities are:

- Systemic hypertension.
- Diabetes mellitus.
- Cardiovascular disease (CVD).

Other risk markers include:

- Obesity and the metabolic syndrome.
- Dyslipidaemia.
- Smoking.
- Social deprivation and poverty.

Many of these factors are identical to those associated with increased CVD risk, highlighting the close association between CKD and CVD (this is discussed further in Chapter 5). Of these, systemic hypertension is the single most important factor predicting the new development of CKD.

Table 8.2 summarizes the findings of some of the community-based studies that have highlighted the links between long-standing hypertension and the development of CKD.

On balance, the evidence suggests that the risk of developing CKD is increased with BP levels considered in the high normal or the pre-hypertensive range (120–139/80–89mmHg).

Hypertension and the risk of progression of CKD

The progression of CKD has been associated with a number of factors, many of which are similar to those that predict the onset

Table 8.2 Community studies linking hypertension to the development of CKD

Study	Country	Population	Follow-up	Findings	Conclusion
Multiple Risk Factor Intervention Trial (MRFIT) (Klag, et al., 1996)	US	332,544 men aged 35–57 years between 1973 and 1975	16 years	Strong, graded relationship between both SBP and DBP with ESRD, independent of age, race, income, smoking, myocardial infarction, and cholesterol.	Compared with men with an optimal level of BP, the relative risk (RR) of ESRD for those with stage 4 hypertension was 22.1. Elevation of BP is a strong independent risk factor for ESRD.
Maryland County Study (Haroun, et al., 2003)	Washington County, US	23,534 men and women	20 years	The adjusted hazard ratio (HR) of developing CKD among women was: 2.5 for normal BP 3.0 for high-normal BP 3.8 for stage 1 hypertension 6.3 for stage 2 hypertension 8.8 for stages 3 or 4 In men, the relationship was similar, but weaker	A large proportion of the attributable risk of CKD in this population was associated with stage 1 hypertension (23%) and cigarette smoking (31%).
Kaiser Permanente database (Hsu, et al., 2005)	California, US	316,675 adults	21 years	The adjusted HR for developing CKD: 1.62 for BP of 120–129/80–85mmHg 1.98 for BP of 130–139/85–89mmHg 2.59 for BP 140–159/90–99mmHg 3.86 for BP of 160–179/100–109mmHg	Even relatively modest elevation in BP is an independent risk factor for CKD.

(Continued)

Table 8.2 (continued) Community studies linking hypertension to the development of CKD

Study	Country	Population	Follow-up	Findings	Conclusion
Atherosclerosis Risk in Communities (ARIC), Cardiovascular Health Study (CHS) (Kshirsagar, et al., 2008)	US	14,155 men and women 45 years or older	9 years	Databases have been pooled to derive a predictive algorithm and scoring system (SCORED) to identify those at risk of CKD within the community.	This analysis has identified hypertension along with diabetes, age, and history of CVD as the major risk factors for future CKD.
Physicians' Health Study (PHS) (Schaeffner, et al., 2008)	Germany	8,093 male participants	14 years	An increase of 10mmHg had corresponding multivariable-adjusted odds ratio (OR) (95% CI) of: 1.11 (1.03–1.19) for SBP 1.11 (1.00–1.23) for MAP 1.14 (1.05–1.25) for PP 1.05 (0.93–1.17) for DBP	Increases in SBP, PP, and MAP were significantly associated with CKD. SBP may be the most clinically useful predictor of CKD.
Okinawa Mass Screening Programme (Tozawa, et al., 2003)	Okinawa, Japan	46,881 men and 51,878 women	17 years	Linked the development of proteinuria and CKD to high baseline levels of blood pressure.	

SBP=systolic blood pressure; DBP=diastolic blood pressure; PP=pulse pressure; MAP=mean arterial pressure; HR=hazard ratio; OR=odds ratio.

of CKD and include both modifiable and non-modifiable factors. Amongst the non-modifiable factors, genetic background, age, gender, and race/ethnicity have been reported to affect the rate of progression of CKD.

Prominent amongst the modifiable risk factors are:

- Systemic hypertension.
- Proteinuria.

Other risk factors that are associated with progression include:

- Dyslipidaemia.
- Obesity.
- Smoking.
- Social deprivation and poverty.

A faster rate of progression of CKD has been associated with raised systolic and diastolic BP as well as elevated pulse pressure. However, a pooled analysis of 11 CKD trials suggested that systolic BP rather than its diastolic counterpart is the most significant determinant of the risk of CKD progression; it reported a progressive increase in the relative risk of progression in those with systolic BP values higher than 120mmHg (Jafar, et al., 2003). Such increased risk was predominantly noted in CKD patients with proteinuria levels >1g/24h, thus highlighting the important interactions between hypertension and proteinuria in determining the risk of progressive CKD.

Causes of hypertension in CKD

Whilst there is abundant evidence linking the development and progression of CKD to systemic hypertension, kidney damage itself is often associated with secondary hypertension, thus initiating a vicious circle of kidney damage, hypertension, and further kidney damage and function decline.

The kidney plays a key role in the regulation of systemic blood pressure. It is involved in the pathogenesis of hypertension and is one of the organs most severely affected by raised blood pressure.

There are a variety of mechanisms of hypertension in CKD which may exist alone or in combination within any one individual. They include:

- Fluid and salt retention and intravascular volume expansion.
- Activation of the renin-angiotensin-aldosterone system (RAAS).
- Activation of the sympathetic nervous system (SNS).
- Activation of the endothelin system.
- Suppression of the nitric oxide axis.
- Vascular stiffness and atherosclerosis.
- Atherosclerotic renovascular disease and renal ischaemia.

Guidelines for the management of hypertension

Timing and target for hypertension management

Global guidelines for the management of essential hypertension agree on a number of points. These include the threshold of initiation of antihypertensive therapy based on risk stratification. In general, it is acceptable to consider those at increased CVD risk for earlier treatment. High risk is defined as a >20% CVD event risk over ten years, which is equivalent to a coronary heart disease (CHD) risk of approximately 10% over ten years. This is pertinent to CKD patients as they are often considered at high CVD risk (see Chapter 5).

A number of specialist societies including KDOQI (US), NICE (UK), CARI (Australasia), and CSN (Canadian) have all recommended targets below 130/80mmHg with established disease, with some recommending lower targets in those with heavy proteinuria.

These recommendations have been based on systematic reviews of the literature featuring a a pooled analysis of 11 large, randomized CKD trials involving 1,860 patients as well as a number of key observational and intervention trials (Table 8.4):

- Modification of Diet in Renal Disease (MDRD) study.
- Second Ramipril Efficacy in Nephropathy (REIN)-2 trial.
- African American Study of Kidney Disease and Hypertension (AASK).
- United Kingdom Prospective Diabetes Study (UKPDS).

Table 8.3 Target BP control recommendations

Society	Recommendations
JNCVII (Chobanian, et al., 2003)	Treating SBP and DBP to targets <140/90mmHg to decrease CVD and renal morbidity and mortality in the general population In patients with diabetes and hypertension or CKD: target BP <130/80mmHg
EBPG (European Society of Hypertension–European Society of Cardiology Guidelines Committee, 2003)	General population: target BP <140/90mmHg General population and high CVD risk: target BP <130/80mmHg
BHS (Williams, et al., 2004)	Threshold for intervention: BP ≥140/90mmHg in high CVD risk individuals, including: CKD: target BP <130/80mmHg CKD + proteinuria >1g/24h: target BP <125/75mmHg
KDOQI (KDOQI, 2004)	CKD: target BP <130/80mmHg CKD with heavy proteinuria as well as diabetic CKD: lower target
NICE hypertension guidelines 2006 (Lewis, 2006)	CKD: target SBP <140mmHg (range 139–120); DBP <90mmHg CKD and diabetes or with proteinuria >1g/24h: target systolic <130mmHg (range 129–120) and diastolic <80mmHg
NICE CKD guidelines 2008 (Crowe, et al., 2008)	CKD: target BP <1380/80mmHg CKD + urine PCR >100mg/mmol: target BP <125/75mmHg
CARI (Harris, et al., 2006)	CKD and proteinuria <0.25g/24h: target BP <130/85mmHg CKD and proteinuria =0.25–1g/24h : target BP <130/80mmHg CKD and proteinuria>1g/24h: target BP <125/75mmHg
CSN (Levin, et al., 2008)	CKD : target BP <130/80mmHg CKD + diabetes: target BP <130/80mmHg

JNCVII=the seventh report of the Joint National Committee for the Prevention, Detection, Evaluation and Treatment of High Blood Pressure; BHS=British Hypertension Society; EBPG=European Best Practice Guidelines for the management of hypertension; KDOQI=Kidney/Disease Outcomes Quality Initiative; NICE=UK National Institute of Health and Clinical Excellence; CARI=Caring for Australasians with Renal Impairment; CSN=Canadian Society of Nephrology

- Appropriate Blood Pressure Control in Diabetes (ABCD) trial.
- Hypertension Optimal Treatment (HOT).
- Heart Outcomes Prevention Evaluation (HOPE) and MICRO-HOPE.

Table 8.4 Summary of intervention studies in hypertension

Trial	Population	Intervention	Achieved BP(mmHg)	Conclusions and recommendations
MDRD (Peterson, et al., 1995)	840 patients with various causes of non-diabetic CKD	MAP: 92 mmHg vs 107mmHg	125/75 135/85	For patients with proteinuria >1g/day: target BP of 125/75. For patients with proteinuria of 0.25 to 1.0g/day: target BP of 130/80 is advisable.
REIN-2 (Ruggenenti, et al., 2005)	335 patients with non-diabetic proteinuric nephropathies receiving background ACEi therapy. Follow-up~1.6 years	Conventional BP control vs intensified BP control	134/82 130/80	No additional benefit in slowing CKD progression from further BP reduction using felodipine.
AASK (Wright, et al., 2002)	1,094 African Americans with hypertensive CKD. Follow-up=5 years	Ramipril: reduced proteinuria (−20%) Metoprolol: reduced proteinuria (−14%) Amlodipine: increased proteinuria (+58%)	Lower BP group 128/78 Usual BP group 141/85	No advantage to further BP reduction; patients with mean BP of 128/78mmHg experienced renal deterioration at the same rate as those achieving a mean of 141/85mmHg.
UKPDS (UKPDS, 1998)	1,148 patients with type2 DM. Follow-up ~10 years	Tight BP control (<150/85mmHg) vs less tight BP control (<180/105mmHg)	144/82 154/87	Those who achieved a tighter BP control had 32% less diabetes-related death and 44% less strokes.
ABCD (Schrier, et al., 2007)	950 patients with type 2 DM and CKD. Follow-up=5.3 years	Intensive BP control vs moderate BP control	132/78 132/86	Those who achieved lower BP had decreased mortality. Less myocardial infarction in those on ACEi. Intensive BP was associated with a reduction of albuminuria. No difference in progression of nephropathy between intensive and moderate BP control.

MDRD=Modification of Diet in Renal Disease study; REIN=Ramipril Efficacy in Nephropathy study; AASK=African American Study of Kidney Disease and Hypertension trial; ABCD=Appropriate Blood Pressure Control in Diabetes study; ACEi=angiotensin-converting enzyme inhibitor

A pooled analysis of 11 major CKD studies (n=1,860) hinted that systolic BP control was more relevant than diastolic in terms of reducing the relative risk of CKD progression. This analysis noted that patients with systolic BP values of <110mmHg were at risk of increased CKD progression (Jafar, et al., 2003). Such a possible J-shaped curve had not previously been reported in relation to the risk of CKD progression with some suggesting that the lower the MAP, the slower the rate of CKD progression in diabetic and non-diabetic CKD (Bakris, et al., 2000).

CKD patients also appear to have a J-shaped relationship with stroke outcomes such that those with systolic BP <120mmHg were at significantly increased risk compared with individuals with CKD and systolic BP of 120–129mmHg (HR 2.51; 95% CI 1.30–4.87); risk increased for BP >130mmHg in CKD (Weiner, et al., 2007).

In general, it is acknowledged that patients with CKD are considered at the highest CVD risk, thus warranting a low threshold for the initiation of antihypertensive treatment and lower target levels. Regarding target BP levels, therefore, it is important to consider levels that would minimize CVD morbidity and mortality. Whilst this has not been directly addressed in CKD patients, the results of large studies aimed at patients at high CVD risk are informative.

The HOT study randomized 18,790 hypertensive individuals into one of three diastolic BP levels (<90mmHg, <85mmHg, and <80mmHg) to determine the impact on incident CVD over a follow-up period of 3.8 years. It showed that for each 5mmHg decrease in diastolic BP, there was a significant reduction in cardiovascular events (Hansson, et al., 1998). In diabetics at high CVD risk, every 2mmHg reduction in systolic BP was associated with a 7% reduction in CHD and a 10% reduction in stroke. In this trial, a diastolic BP value of 85mmHg appeared to reduce the risk of major cardiovascular events by 27% with no further improvement at lower DBP levels (80mmHg). However, a post hoc analysis of 470 individual with a serum creatinine >133micromol/L showed no difference in cardiovascular events rate between the three BP groups.

A post hoc analysis of the HOPE study suggested a CVD benefit associated with ACE inhibition with ramipril in non-proteinuric CKD patients. However, concerns were expressed when this trial was reviewed and a dissociation of the antihypertensive effect of ramipril from its cardioprotective effect was not shown (Onuigbo, 2008).

Targeting proteinuria

Microalbuminuria, overt albuminuria, and proteinuria are well-known markers associated with diabetic and non-diabetic CKD. Microalbuminuria refers to levels of albumin in the urine detected below thresholds for usual dipstick proteinuria; it is not a different molecule or type of albumin. Importantly, thresholds have been established for health and in specific circumstances. Sustained microalbuminuria (more than one of three samples) represents significant abnormalities. Recent data suggest a high prevalence of microalbuminuria in the general population. Microalbuminuria has also been linked to increased CVD risk. Proteinuria is a well-established, poor prognostic marker for CKD progression.

Microalbuminuria is present in a variety of conditions other than CKD, including:

- Older age (usually in the presence of other comorbidities).
- Obesity.
- Hypertension.
- Diabetes.
- CVD.
- Chronic inflammatory conditions, including dermatitis (psoriasis), arthritis, chronic hepatitis, and inflammatory bowel disease.
- Smoking.
- Post-exercise/strenuous activity.

A growing body of evidence points to the fact that microalbuminuria may, therefore, be more a marker of chronic inflammation and/or endothelial dysfunction rather than progressive CKD. Microalbuminuria is highly predictive of CVD; this is not surprising since it is thought to be a reliable marker of diffuse vascular stiffness and damage.

In contrast, overt albuminuria/proteinuria (such as can be detected using conventional dipstick), along with hypertension, is a very significant risk marker of progressive CKD. In fact, some studies suggested that the beneficial impact of proteinuria reduction is greater and independent from that of hypertension.

As mentioned above, the risk of CKD progression is determined by the severity of proteinuria with those with urine protein levels <1g/24h having a low risk, even when BP levels are elevated. By contrast, CKD patients with proteinuria >1g/24h have an increased risk of decline of kidney function, even at high normal levels of systolic BP (Jafar, et al., 2003). Therefore, it is imperative to aim to reduce 24-hour urinary protein excretion to levels below 1g. This should be attempted even after BP target levels have been achieved. There is considerable evidence to suggest that the inhibition of the RAAS is a very effective way of reducing proteinuria in diabetic nephropathies and proteinuric CKD.

Management of hypertension in CKD

The management of systemic hypertension in CKD includes lifestyle modifications as well as pharmacological interventions.

Lifestyle modifications in CKD

These follow the same recommendations made to patients with essential hypertension, encouraging dietary salt reduction and regular exercise (Table 8.5). Of note, dietary salt restriction has a synergistic antihypertensive effect when combined with ACEis/ARBs.

Table 8.5 Lifestyle modifications for the management of hypertension

Intervention	Recommendations
Weight reduction	Maintain ideal BMI (20–25kg/m^2)
DASH eating plan	Consume diet rich in fruit, vegetables, low-fat dairy products with reduced content of saturated and total fat
Dietary sodium restriction	Reduce dietary sodium intake to 100mmol/day (<2.4g sodium or <6g sodium chloride)
Alcohol moderation	Men ≤21 units per week; women ≤14 units per week
Smoking	Cessation of smoking
Physical activity	Engage in regular aerobic physical activity, e.g. brisk walking for at least 30min most days

DASH=Dietary Approaches to Stop Hypertension

Pharmacological interventions

These are invariably necessary for the control of hypertension in CKD. Inhibition of the RAAS by ACEis or ARBs has been favoured for the initial management of diabetic and proteinuric, non-diabetic CKD, based on the above data and the recommendations of a number of guidelines on the management of hypertensive CKD.

Table 8.6 Management of hypertension in CKD guidelines

Organization	Recommendations
KDOQI guidelines (KDOQI, 2004)	Diabetic CKD: ACEi/ARB preferentially
	Other agents to reduce CVD risk and reach BP target: diuretic preferred, then beta-blocker or calcium channel blocker
	Non-diabetic CKD with urine PCR >200mg/g: same as diabetic CKD
	Non-diabetic CKD with urine PCR <200mg/g: none preferred
	Other agents to reduce CVD risk and reach BP target: diuretic preferred, then ACEi, ARB, beta-blocker or calcium channel blocker
	CKD in the transplant recipient: none preferred
	Other agents to reduce CVD risk and reach BP target: calcium channel blocker, diuretic, beta-blocker, ACEi, ARB
NICE CKD guideline (Crowe, et al., 2008)	Diabetic CKD: preferentially started with ACEi/ARB
	CKD + hypertension + proteinuria >0.5g/24h or ACR> 30mg/mmol): preferentially started on an ACEi/ARB
	CKD + proteinuria (>1g/24h) without hypertension: preferentially started on ACEi/ARB [2]
The Scottish Intercollegiate Guidelines Network (SIGN, 2008)	CKD + proteinuria >1g/24h: preferentially start with ACEi/ARB
CARI (Harris, et al., 2006)	ACEis and ARBs are more effective than others in slowing diabetic and non-diabetic CKD
CSN (Levin, et al., 2008)	CKD with proteinuria (proteinuria >0.5g/24h or ACR >30mg/mmol): treatment should include ACEi or ARB
	Non-proteinuric CKD (ACR <30mg/mmol): choice of anti-hypertensive agent

NICE=National Institute of Health and Clinical Excellence (UK); KDOQI=Kidney Disease Outcomes Quality Initiative; SIGN=Scottish Intercollegiate Guidelines Network; CARI=Caring for Australasians with Renal Impairment; CSN=Canadian Society of Nephrology; ACEi=angiotensin converting enzyme inhibitor; ARB=angiotensin receptor blocker

Meta-analyses of major CKD trials have suggested that the blockade of the RAAS is beneficial when proteinuria levels exceed 1g/24h (Jafar, et al., 2003), although a more recent analysis suggested that such benefit may be extended to CKD patients with proteinuria above 0.5g/24h (Kent, et al., 2007).

However, it is important to appreciate that most analyses showing superiority of ACEis and ARBs over other antihypertensive agents in CKD have been confined to patients with diabetic kidney disease or those with proteinuric, non-diabetic CKD. For instance, the REIN pivotal studies of ACE inhibition's impact on the progression of non-diabetic CKD failed to show a benefit in patients with proteinuria <1.5–3g/24h.

Also, most studies failed to fully dissociate the beneficial effect of ACEis and ARBs on CKD progression from their superior BP control effect (Griffin & Bidani, 2006).

Finally, the indiscriminate use of ACEi/ARBs in CKD patients is not without risks. It is well known that patients with renovascular disease and ischaemic nephropathy may be at risk of further renal dysfunction when using these agents.

It is generally accepted that up to 30% acute increase in serum creatinine or a fall in GFR of less than 25% within a week of initiation of ACEi/ARBs in patients with CKD is acceptable and predictable. However, close and prolonged monitoring is warranted as some patients continue to have a rise in serum creatinine within the first three months of ACEi/ARB initiation.

Risk stratification of CKD and CVD risk

With the above in mind, what recommendations can be made regarding the management of hypertensive CKD?

The choice of agents in hypertensive CKD may have to take into considerations the presence of other CKD and CVD risk markers:

- Proteinuria.
- Stage of CKD.
- Type of CKD.

- Race and ethnicity.
- Smoking.
- Dyslipidaemia.

Proteinuria

Evidence suggests that ACEis/ARBs are more effective than conventional agents in CKD patients with significant proteinuria (>1g/24h) and MAP levels >110mmHg (BP >140/90mmHg).

This would justify the use of RAAS inhibitors as the initial treatment of choice in diabetic and proteinuric CKD. In such patients, including those with advanced diabetic nephropathy, it has been suggested that dihydropyridine calcium channel blockers (CCB) may not be effective at reducing proteinuria. There may be an advantage for using non-dihydropyridine CCB such as verapamil and diltiazem, as they have been shown in a small number of studies to be as effective as ACEis in reducing proteinuria in patients with type 2 diabetic nephropathy. Beta-blockers have modest, if any, intrinsic anti-proteinuric effect.

To control proteinuria, ACEis/ARBs treatment is often ineffective unless combined with dietary salt restriction (below Na 100mmol/day, i.e. <2.4g sodium or <6g sodium chloride) and diuretic therapy.

As the initial one to six months of proteinuria reduction effect determines long-term outcome, it is sensible to aim at maximal suppression of proteinuria, aiming for values <1g/24h; for that, the combination of an ACEi and ARB may be justifiable.

The evidence for an additional advantage for combination therapy remains controversial. The COOPERATE study in non-diabetic CKD showed that ACEis and ARBs have additive anti-proteinuric effects independently of their BP lowering impact (Nakao, et al., 2003). The combination led to a beneficial effect on the progression of CKD as a function of the reduction of proteinuria and independently of BP levels. However, this study has been severely criticized. More recently, data from the ONTARGET study of patients with CVD implied a faster rate of progression of CKD in patients treated with a combination of ramipril and telmisartan, thus raising some concern over such a combination in patients with CVD and impaired renal function (Mann, et al., 2008).

Stage of CKD

There is little doubt that the initial level of GFR at the initiation of treatment affects prognosis with patients with CKD stages 3 to 5 at higher risk. Most data evaluating the impact of antihypertensives on the progression of CKD have focused on these patients with the highest risk of progression, where changes in BP levels and proteinuria have detectable impacts on CKD progression over short observation times.

Patients with CKD stages 3 and 4 and heavy proteinuria would benefit from ACEis/ARBs as discussed above with a target BP <125/75mmHg. It has also been argued that even those with CKD stage 5 would benefit; this awaits further confirmation and warrants caution as these agents could easily precipitate irreversible ESRD.

In patients with CKD stages 1 and 2 with mild proteinuria (<1g/24h), progression is often slow and there is little evidence that progression is affected by the type of antihypertensive agent used. There is also a paucity of data on their CVD risk in the absence of decreased GFR (<60mL/min) and/or anaemia. Therefore, in these patients, it would be reasonable to apply the risk stratification recommendations drawn for the treatment of essential hypertension:

- High CVD risk: 20% chance of an events over a 10-year period:
- Those with age >55 years, male gender, smokers, and hyperlipidaemia and/or a family history of CVD should be treated early (BP= 140/90mmHg) and BP levels should be reduced to <130/80mmHg (Chobanian, et al., 2003).
- Low CVD risk patients: target BP levels of 140/90mmHg would be acceptable, bearing in mind their low CKD and CVD risk.

The guidelines on the treatment of hypertension in the general population issued by NICE (Lewis, 2006) suggest that the initiation of antihypertensive therapy with a thiazide diuretic and/or a calcium antagonist would be a reasonable and cost-effective first choice in those over the age of 55 and black patients of any age. These agents seem to provide better cardiovascular risk reduction than beta-blockers, in particular against stroke, and are marginally more cost-effective than ACEis/ARBs. This choice is based on a meta-analysis of major hypertension clinical trials as well as a formal economic evaluation. They recommend ACEis as first-line treatment in hypertensive patients younger than 55 years. If more than two agents need to be used to control BP, they recommend a combination of diuretic, calcium antagonist, and ACEi/ARB.

A UK CKD consensus meeting (Williams & Rodger, 2007) suggested that for most patients with early CKD (stages 1 to 3) without significant proteinuria (<1g/24h or urinary PCR <100mg/mmol), the primary objective of treatment is to reduce the risk of stroke and heart disease with the choice of antihypertensive agents according to national guidelines. These recommendations agree with those of the British Hypertension Society and take into consideration the absence of evidence of an additional renoprotective effect of angiotensin inhibitors in non-proteinuric CKD.

Type of CKD

Patients with diabetic nephropathy should preferentially be treated by initial inhibition of the RAAS; there is no evidence of a difference in efficacy between ACEis and ARBs in these patients. In non-diabetic CKD patients, the stage of CKD and proteinuria should be the major determinant of choice of antihypertensive agent rather than the nature of the underlying nephropathy. In a number of chronic glomerulonephritis, including membranous and IgA nephropathy, ACEis have been shown to be effective at reducing proteinuria and slowing the progression of renal insufficiency. In patients with polycystic kidney disease, it has been argued that ACEis are both beneficial and detrimental; this may reflect the stage of CKD with an early intervention having a more beneficial effect.

An increasing number of patients are recognized as having renovascular disease. These also include a proportion of type 2 diabetic patients with CKD. It is imperative to have a high index of suspicion of such patients in the face of a disproportionally high systolic BP and a wide pulse pressure in patients with a history of atherosclerotic vascular disease. ACEis and ARBs should be avoided in these patients as they can precipitate further deterioration in renal function as the ischaemic kidney depends to a large extent on angiotensin II-mediated, efferent, arteriolar vasoconstriction to maintain the capillary pressure and filtration of its hypoperfused glomeruli.

Race and ethnicity

It is generally accepted that black people from African or African Caribbean origin have higher rates of hypertension and higher BP levels than white individuals. This is associated with a higher CKD and CVD risk, with the exception of CHD which is lower than in whites. Hypertension in the black population is often volume-dependent and salt-sensitive, reflecting a low renin status, favouring dietary salt restriction, and diuretic therapy. Among black patients in the ALLHAT study, ACE inhibition led to a significantly higher rate of CVD events; strokes, and congestive heart failure. However, the AASK trial of African American patients with CKD showed ramipril to be superior to amlodipine; the amlodipine arm had to be stopped prematurely because of apparent worsening of CKD. The decision has been controversial because it implied that CCB may not be suitable for black individuals with CKD. In general, it is advisable to treat black patients with CKD along similar lines to their white counterparts, including the inhibition of the RAAS along with dietary salt restriction and vigorous diuretic therapy.

In the US and UK, individuals from Asian origin have a higher prevalence of diabetes mellitus and hypertension as well as renal and cardiovascular complications. British Asians may also have a faster rate of progression of diabetic nephropathy. There is no evidence that these individuals respond differently to antihypertensive agents compared to Caucasians. However, their high susceptibility to glucose intolerance/diabetes, obesity, and dyslipidaemia may affect the choice of antihypertensive agents. With that in mind, agents modifying the RAAS may have therapeutic advantages as they decrease the incidence of diabetes and have beneficial effects on components of the metabolic syndrome.

Smoking

Patients with CKD who are heavy smokers are at an increased risk of progression of diabetic and non-diabetic CKD. It has been shown in one study that ACE inhibition considerably reduced the smoking-associated risk of progression to ESRD (Orth, et al., 1998). Clearly, this warrants confirmation and further investigations.

Dyslipidaemia

The initiation and progression of CKD have been linked to dyslipidaemia. Therefore, this should be taken into consideration when prescribing antihypertensive agents as some such as diuretics and beta-blockers increase serum lipids. Also, CKD patients are at high CVD risk and the control of dyslipidaemia is recommendable in such at-risk group of patients.

A recent meta-analysis has shown that statins significantly reduce lipid concentrations and cardiovascular end points in patients with CKD, irrespective of the stage of the disease, but with no benefit on all-cause mortality (Strippoli, et al., 2008).

Table 8.7 Treatment of hypertension according to risk stratification

Risk stratification	Agent	Target BP
Proteinuria	>1g/24h: ACEi/ARB followed by diuretics, and then non-dihydropyridine CCB (regardless of CKD stage or type)	<125/75mmHg
	<1g/24h: choice of anti-hypertensive agents according to national guidelines	<130/80mmHg
Stage of CKD	CKD stages 1 and 2: high CVD risk	<130/80mmHg
	Low CVD risk	<140/90mmHg
	CKD stages 3, 4, and 5	<130/80mmHg
Type of CKD	Diabetic nephropathy: ACEis or ARBs Renovascular disease: avoid ACEis and ARBs IgA and ADPKD : ACEis are preferable initially	According to CKD stage and proteinuria
Race and ethnicity	No evidence to treat blacks and Asians differently	According to CKD stage and proteinuria
Smoking	ACEis may be preferable according to one study that showed significant protection in smokers (Orth, et al., 1998)	According to CKD stage and proteinuria
Dyslipidaemia	Caution with diuretics and beta-blockers	According to CKD stage and proteinuria

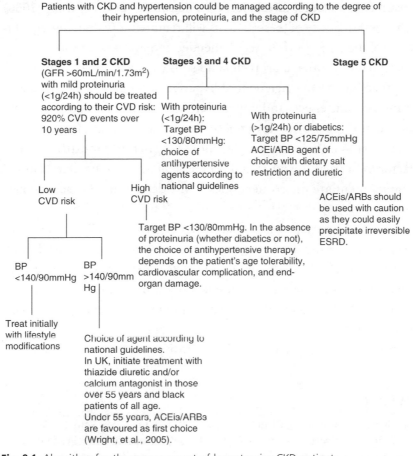

Patients with CKD and hypertension could be managed according to the degree of their hypertension, proteinuria, and the stage of CKD

Stages 1 and 2 CKD
(GFR >60mL/min/1.73m²)
with mild proteinuria
(<1g/24h) should be treated
according to their CVD risk:
920% CVD events over
10 years

Stages 3 and 4 CKD

With proteinuria
(<1g/24h):
  Target BP
  <130/80mmHg:
  choice of
  antihypertensive
  agents according to
  national guidelines

With proteinuria
(>1g/24h) or diabetics:
Target BP <125/75mmHg
ACEi/ARB agent of
choice with dietary salt
restriction and diuretic

Stage 5 CKD

ACEis/ARBs should
be used with caution
as they could easily
precipitate irreversible
ESRD.

Low
CVD risk

High
CVD risk

Target BP <130/80mmHg. In the absence
of proteinuria (whether diabetics or not),
the choice of antihypertensive therapy
depends on the patient's age tolerability,
cardiovascular complication, and end-
organ damage.

BP
<140/90mmHg

BP
>140/90mm
Hg

Treat initially
with lifestyle
modifications

Choice of agent according to
national guidelines.
In UK, initiate treatment with
thiazide diuretic and/or
calcium antagonist in those
over 55 years and black
patients of all age.
Under 55 years, ACEis/ARBs
are favoured as first choice
(Wright, et al., 2005).

Fig. 8.1 Algorithm for the management of hypertensive CKD patients

Conclusion

In conclusion, the management of hypertension in CKD depends on the renal and cardiovascular risk profile of the patient. Patients with low renal and cardiovascular risks, namely those with CKD stages 1 and 2 and no or mild proteinuria (<1g/24h), could be treated according to guidelines set by national and international hypertension societies. On the other hand, those with more advanced renal insufficiency (CKD stages 3–5) and/or those with proteinuria who are at high renal and CVD risks should be treated according to the K/DOQI and NICE guidelines for the management of hypertension in CKD with lower treatment and target thresholds <130/80mmHg (Levey & Uhlig, 2006). The great majority of these patients will require more than one agent to control their BP down to recommended target levels <130/80mmHg. Compliance is often a problem, and so the conventional stepped care approach to the management of hypertension may not be optimal to minimize side effects and improve compliance. Combination therapy of two or three drugs at lower doses may be a better initial option.

Hypertension is the single, most important, modifiable risk factor to prevent the onset and progression of CKD. Its detection and management are the cornerstones of the detection and management of CKD.

It is very important when treating hypertension in CKD to take into consideration the detection and management of all the modifiable factors associated with hypertension such as proteinuria, hyperglycaemia (in diabetes), obesity, dyslipidaemia, and smoking. It is expected that such a multifactorial approach to the management of progressive CKD will not only slow the decline of kidney function, or even halt it, but also minimize the CVD morbidity and mortality associated with CKD.

References

Bakris, G.L., Williams, M., Dworkin, L., Elliott, W.J., Epstein, M., Toto, R., Tuttle, K., Douglas, J., Hsueh, W., Sowers, J., 2000. Preserving renal function in adults with hypertension and diabetes: a consensus approach. *American Journal of Kidney Diseases*, 36(3), pp.646–61.

Chobanian, A.V., Bakris, G.L., Black, H.R., Cushman, W.C., Green, L.A., Izzo, J.L.Jr, Jones, D.W., Materson, B.J., Oparil, S., Wright, J.T., Jr, Roccella, E.J.; Joint National Committee on prevention, detection, evaluation, and treatment of high blood pressure. National Heart Lung, and Blood Institute; National High Blood Pressure Education Programme Coordinating Committee, 2003. Seventh report of the joint national committee on prevention, detection, evaluation, and treatment of high blood pressure. *Hypertension*, 42(6), pp.1206–52.

Crowe, E., Halpin, D., Stevens, P., 2008. Early identification and management of chronic kidney disease: summary of NICE guidance. *British Medical Journal*, 337, p.a1530.

European Society of Hypertension–European Society of Cardiology Guidelines Committee, 2003. 2003 European Society of Hypertension–European Society of Cardiology guidelines for the management of arterial hypertension. *Journal of Hypertension*, 21(6), pp.1011–53.

Griffin, K.A., Bidani, A.K., 2006. Progression of renal disease: renoprotective specificity of renin-angiotensin system blockade. *Clinical Journal of the American Society of Nephrology*, 1(5), pp.1054–65.

Hansson, L., Zanchetti, A., Carruthers, S.G., Dahlof, B., Elmfeldt, D., Julius, S., Menard, J., Rahn, K.H., Wedel, H., Westerling, S., 1998. Effects of intensive blood-pressure lowering and low-dose aspirin in patients with hypertension: principal results of the Hypertension Optimal Treatment (HOT) randomised trial. *Lancet*, 351(9118), pp.1755–62.

Haroun, M.K., Jaar, B.G., Hoffman, S.C., Comstock, G.W., Klag, M.J., Coresh, J., 2003. Risk factors for chronic kidney disease: a prospective study of 23,534 men and women in Washington County, Maryland. *Journal of the American Society of Nephrology*, 14, pp.2934–41.

Harris, D., Thomas, M., Johnson, D., Nicholls, K., Gillin, A., Caring for Australasians, with Renal Impairment (CARI), 2006. The CARI guidelines. Prevention of progression of kidney disease. *Nephrology (Carlton)*, 11(Suppl 1), S2–197.

Hsu, C.Y., McCulloch, C.E., Darbinian, J., Go, A.S., Iribarren, C., 2005. Elevated blood pressure and risk of end-stage renal disease in subjects without baseline kidney disease. *Archives of Internal Medicine*, 165(8), pp.923–8.

Jafar, T.H., Stark, P.C., Schmid, C.H., Landa, M., Maschio, G., de Jong, P.E., de Zeeuw, D., Shahinfar, S., Toto, R., Levey, A.S.; AIPRD Study Group, 2003. Progression of chronic kidney disease: the role of blood pressure control, proteinuria, and angiotensin-converting enzyme inhibition: a patient-level meta-analysis. *Annals of Internal Medicine*, 139(4), pp.244–52.

KDOQI, 2002. Clinical practice guidelines for chronic kidney disease: evaluation, classification, and stratification. *American Journal of Kidney Diseases*, 39(Suppl 2), S7–266.

KDOQI, 2004. Clinical practice guidelines on hypertension and antihypertensive agents in chronic kidney disease. *American Journal of Kidney Diseases*, 43(Suppl 1) (5), S1–290.

Kent, D.M., Jafar, T.H., Hayward, R.A., Tighiourt, H., Landa, M., de Jong, P., de Zeeuw, D., Remuzzi, G., Kamper, A.L., Levey, A.S., 2007. Progression risk, urinary protein excretion, and treatment effects of angiotensin-converting enzyme inhibitors in nondiabetic kidney disease. *Journal of the American Society of Nephrology*, 18(6), pp.1959–65.

Kshirsagar, A.V., Bang, H., Bomback, A.S., Vupputuri, S., Shoham, D.A., Kern, L.M., Klemmer, P.J., Mazumbar, M., August, P.A., 2008. A simple algorithm to predict incident kidney disease. *Archives of Internal Medicine*, 168(22), pp.2466–73.

Levey, A.S., Uhlig, K., 2006. Which antihypertensive agents in chronic kidney disease? *Annals of Internal Medicine*, 144(3), pp,213–5.

Levin, A., Hemmelgarn, B., Culleton, B., Tobe, S., McFarlane, P., Ruzicka, M., Burns, K., Manns, B., White, C., Madore, F., Moist, L., Klarenbach, S., Barrett, B., Foley, R., Jindal, K., Senior, P., Pannu, N., Shurraw, S., Akbari, A., Cohn, A., Reslerova, M., Deved, V., Mendelssohn, D., Nesrallah, G., Kappel, J., Tonelli, M.; Canadian

Society of Nephrology, 2008. Guidelines for the management of chronic kidney disease. *Canadian Medical Association Journal*, 179(11), pp.1154–62.

Lewis, P.S., 2006. The NICE hypertension guideline update 2006: a welcome revision. *British Journal of Hospital Medicine (London)*, 67(9), pp.454–5.

Lewis, J., Phillips, R.A., Toto, R.D., Middleton, J.P., Rostand, S.G., African American Study of Kidney Disease and Hypertension Study Group, 2002. Effect of blood pressure lowering and antihypertensive drug class on progression of hypertensive kidney disease. *Journal of American Medical Association*, 288(19), pp.2421–31.

Mann, J.F., Schmieder, R.E., McQueen, M., Dyal, L., Schumacher, H., Pogue, J., Wang, X., Maggioni, A., Budaj, A., Chaithiraphan, S., Dickstein, K., Keltai, M., Metsarinne, K., Oto, A., Parkhomenko, A., Piegas, L.S., Svendsen, T.L., Teo, K.K., Yusuf, S., ONTARGET investigators, 2008. Renal outcomes with telmisartan, ramipril, or both, in people at high vascular risk (the ONTARGET study): a multicentre, randomised, double-blind, controlled trial. *Lancet*, 372(9638), pp.547–53.

Nakao, N., Yoshimura, A., Morita, H., Takada, M., Kayano, T., Ideura, T., 2003. Combination treatment of angiotensin-II receptor blocker and angiotensin-converting-enzyme inhibitor in non-diabetic renal disease (COOPERATE): a randomised controlled trial. *Lancet*, 361(9352), pp.117–24.

Onuigbo, M.A., 2009. Reno-prevention vs. reno-protection: a critical re-appraisal of the evidence-base from the large RAAS blockade trials after ontarget--a call for more circumspection. QJM, 102(3), pp.155–67.Klag, M.J., Whelton, P.K., Randall, B.L., Neaton, J.D., Brancati, F.L., Ford, C.E., Shulman, N.B., Stamler, J., 1996. Blood pressure and end-stage renal disease in men. *New England Journal of Medicine*, 334(1), pp.13–8.

Orth, S.R., Stockmann, A., Conradt, C., Ritz, E., Ferro, M., Kreusser, W., Piccoli, G., Rambausek, M., Roccatello, D., Schafer, K., Sieberth, H.G., Wanner, C., Watschinger, B., Zucchelli, P., 1998. Smoking as a risk factor for end-stage renal failure in men with primary renal disease. *Kidney International*, 54(3), pp.926–31.

Peterson, J.C., Adler, S., Burkart, J.M., Greene, T., Hebert, L.A., Hunsicker, L.G., King, A.J., Klahr, S., Massry, S.G., Seifter, J.L., 1995. Blood pressure control, proteinuria, and the progression of renal disease: the Modification of Diet in Renal Disease Study. *Annals of Internal Medicine*, 123(10), pp.754–62.

Ruggenenti, P., Perna, A., Loriga, G., Ganeva, M., Ene–Iordache, B., Turturro, M., Lesti, M., Perticucci, E., Chakarski, I.N., Leonardis, D., Garini, G., Sessa, A., Basile, C., Alpa, M., Scanziani, R., Sorba, G., Zoccali, C., Remuzzi, G., REIN-2 Study Group, 2005. Blood pressure control for renoprotection in patients with non-diabetic chronic renal disease (REIN-2): multicentre, randomized controlled trial. *Lancet*, 365(9463), pp.939–46.

Schaeffner, E.S., Kurth, T., Bowman, T.S., Gelber, R.P., Gaziano, J.M., 2008. Blood pressure measures and risk of chronic kidney disease in men. *Nephrology Dialysis Transplantation*, 23(4), pp.1246–51.

Schrier, R.W., Estacio, R.O., Mehler, P.S., Hiatt, W.R., 2007. Appropriate blood pressure control in hypertensive and normotensive type 2 diabetes mellitus: a summary of the ABCD trial. *Nature Clinical Practice Nephrology*, 3(8), pp.428–38.

Scottish Intercollegiate Guidelines Network (SIGN) CKD Guidelines, Guideline No. 103, ISBN 9781905813308, June 2008. Website: http://www.sign.ac.uk/ guidelines/fulltext/103/index.html

Strippoli, G.F., Navaneethan, S.D., Johnson, D.W., Perkovic, V., Pellegrini, F., Nicolucci, A., Craig, J.C., 2008. Effects of statins in patients with chronic kidney disease: meta-analysis and meta-regression of randomised controlled trials. *British Medical Journal*, 336(7645), pp.645–51.

Tozawa, M., Iseki, K, Iseki, C., Kinjo, K., Ikemiya, Y., Takishita., S., 2003. Blood pressure predicts risk of developing end-stage renal disease in men and women. *Hypertension*, 41(6), pp.1341–5.

UK Prospective Diabetes Study Group, 1998. Efficacy of atenolol and captopril in reducing risk of macrovascular and microvascular complications in type 2 diabetes: UKPDS 39. *British Medical Journal*, 317(7160), pp.713–20.

Weiner, D.E., Tighiouart, H., Levey, A.S., Elsayed, E., Griffith, J.L., Salem, D.N., Sarnak, M.J., 2007. Lowest systolic blood pressure is associated with stroke in stages 3 to 4 chronic kidney disease. *Journal of the American Society of Nephrology*, 18(3), pp.960–6.

Williams, B., Poulter, N.R., Brown, M.J., Davis, M., McInnes, G.T., Potter, J.F., Sever, P.S., McG Thom, S; British Hypertension Society, 2004. Guidelines for management of hypertension: report of the fourth working party of the British Hypertension Society, 2004—BHS IV. *Journal of Human Hypertension*, 18(3), pp.139–85.

Williams, B., Rodger, S.C., 2007. Consensus conference on early chronic kidney disease. *Nephrology Dialysis Transplantation*, 22(Suppl 9), ix1–63.

Wright, J.T., Bakris, G., Greene, T., Agodoa, L.Y., Appel, L.J., Charleston, J., Cheek, D., Douglas–Baltimore, J.G., Gassman, J., Glassock, R., Hebert, L., Jamerson, K., Lewis, J., Phillips, R.A., Toto, R.D., Middleton, J.P., Rostand, S.G., African American Study of Kidney Disease and Hypertension Study Group, 2002. Effect of blood pressure lowering and antihypertensive drug class on progression of hypertensive kidney disease: results from the AASK trial. *Journal of the American Medical Association*, 288(19), 2421–31.

Wright, J.T., Dunn, J.K., Cutler, J.A., Davis, B.R., Cushman, W.C., Ford, C.E., Haywood, L.J., Leenen, F.H., Margolis, K.L., Papademetriou, V., Probstfield, J.L., Whelton, P.K., Habib, G.B.; ALLHAT Collaborative Research Group, 2005. Outcomes in hypertensive black and nonblack patients treated with chlorthalidone, amlodipine, and lisinopril. *Journal of the Americal Medical Association*, 293(13), pp.1595–608.

Chapter 9

Clinical strategies for the management of chronic kidney disease complications: perspectives for primary care

Monica Beaulieu, Neil Boudville, and Adeera Levin

Overview and perspective: complications of chronic kidney disease

Chronic kidney disease (CKD) is associated with a myriad of complications, both due to reduced kidney function itself and/or as a consequence of the conditions that may have caused CKD such as diabetes and cardiovascular disease (CVD). Much of the morbidity and mortality of CKD is due to CVD, which is covered more extensively in Chapter 4 of this text.

The purpose of this chapter is to identify complications specific to CKD and to outline strategies for their management. Given the increasing awareness by physicians of the prevalence of CKD, it is critical to ensure that basic strategies to address complications are implemented at early stages of the disease to reduce associated morbidity and mortality.

The management of the following key complications will be discussed and are summarized in Tables 9.1 and 9.2:

- CVD (more extensively covered in Chapter 4).
- Anaemia.
- Bone and mineral metabolism.
- Metabolic acidosis.
- Malnutrition.

In addition, the treatment options for patients with end-stage renal disease (ESRD) will be discussed, including:

- Kidney transplantation.
- Dialysis.
  - Haemodialysis.
  - Peritoneal dialysis.
- Comprehensive conservative care.

CVD in CKD

Individuals with CKD are at increased cardiovascular risk. Traditional risk factors (hypertension, diabetes, metabolic abnormalities) explain some, but not all, of this increased risk. CKD is considered a 'disease multiplier' for CVD, meaning that patients with CKD and a traditional cardiovascular risk factor have a much higher rate of cardiovascular events. In fact, the majority of patients with CKD do not progress to ESRD, but rather die from a cardiovascular cause. Therefore, close attention to the treatment of cardiovascular risk factors is absolutely essential in CKD patients and forms one of the mainstays of therapy.

Causes

- The aetiology is multifactorial, reflecting the complex interaction of many factors.
- Many CKD complications (anaemia, abnormalities of bone and mineral metabolism, metabolic acidosis, malnutrition) may also negatively impact on cardiovascular health and fitness levels.

Treatment strategies (Table 9.1)

- The use of low dose aspirin (e.g. ASA 81mg daily) is recommended for cardiovascular protection.
- Cardiovascular risk profile assessment and modification, including smoking cessation.
- Treatment of hypertension (target BP to <130/80).
  - Usually requires at least three medications (diuretic, ACEi/ARB, calcium channel blocker or beta-blocker).

Table 9.1 Overview of the objectives of the general care for CKD and its complications**

Care	Objective	Target
Hypertension	Measure and record at diagnosis and at every visit thereafter.	BP <130/80mmHg Use of ACEis or ARBs for proteinuric CKD
Dyslipidaemia	A fasting lipid profile should be measured in adults with CKD stages 1–3 and adults with CKD stage 4 if the results would influence the decision to initiate or alter lipid-modifying treatment.	Initiation and targets for CKD stages 1–3 are as per the general population. CKD stage 4 LDL-cholesterol <2.0mmol/L and total cholesterol: HDL ratio <4.0
Diabetes	Glycaemic control should be part of a multifactorial intervention strategy addressing BP control and cardiovascular risk.	HbA1c ≤7.0% (0.07)
Lifestyle management	Record weight and BMI at each visit for comparison.	Maintenance of BMI 18.5–24.9kg/m². Waist circumference <102cm for men and <88cm for women
Smoking	Encourage patient to stop; enquire at every visit.	Complete cessation
Proteinuria	Screening for proteinuria (spot urine for ACR) in all patients who are at high risk of kidney disease.	Adults with diabetes and persistent albuminuria (ACR >2.0mg/mmol in males, >2.8mg/mmol in females) should receive an ACEi or ARB to delay the progression of CKD, even in the absence of hypertension.
Assessment of conditions associated with CKD	Measure mineral metabolism, haematology and nutrition profiles at least yearly, more frequently with advanced kidney disease.	Anaemia: Hb 110g/L (range 100–120g/L) Transferrin sat >20%, ferritin >100ng/mL Bone disease: calcium and phosphate levels within normal range Nutrition and acidosis: albumin >35g/L; bicarbonate >22mmol/L
Preparation for RRT	Ensure education about all modality options is available. Preserve veins in patients who may need vascular access creation.	Referral to multidisciplinary care team if GFR <30mL/min or evidence of progression
Conservative management and end-of-life care	Ensure access to multidisciplinary care team with tools to deal with end-of-life issues.	Dignified and supported dying process accessed by all

** Adapted with permission from British Columbia Guidelines and Protocols Advisory Committee (BCGPAC)

Table 9.2 Objectives and strategies for specific complications of CKD

Parameter	Objective and rationale	Target	Suggested treatments
Haemoglobin	Measure and record; follow trend and reticulocyte count. Initial evaluation and if changes: assess iron stores (transferrin sat, ferritin). Rule out additional causes (folate, B12, protein electrophoresis), if indicated. Regular review, depending on stage and treatment.	Hb 110–120g/L on therapy Normal if no therapy Transferrin sat >20 Ferritin >100	Iron replacement (oral or IV) ESAs
PTH	Measure under same conditions and at same laboratory at least 6-monthly. Discuss with specialist for optimal treatment strategies.	Set patient specific goals	Dietary phosphate restriction Vitamin D therapy Calcimimetic therapies
Calcium	Avoid hypo- or hypercalcaemia	Normal laboratory values	Calcium supplementation
Phosphate	Avoid hypo- or hyperphosphataemia and malnutrition	Normal laboratory values	Dietary phosphate restriction Binders: aluminium hydroxide, calcium carbonate, Sevalamer, Lanthanum
Serum bicarbonate	Avoid persistent metabolic acidosis (malnutrition, stone formation, resistance to vitamin D)	>22mmol/L	Sodium bicarbonate or calcium carbonate Dietary counselling

- For patients with proteinuric kidney disease (diabetic and non-diabetic), the therapy should include an ACEi, or ARB, or both.
- Treat comorbidities that contribute to vascular risk (optimal blood sugar control in diabetics):
  - HbA1c target <7%.
- Treatment of hyperlipidaemia (diet and lipid-lowering medications) as required.
- Smoking cessation.

The heterogeneous nature of the CKD population, as well as their exclusion from many clinical trials, leads to difficulties in extrapolating from the general population or to specific stages of CKD. Given the prevalence of CKD in the general population, especially at relatively earlier stages, the current clinical judgement would suggest that treatments should be similar to those at high cardiovascular risk.

Furthermore, CVD may arise before, with, or as a consequence of CKD, and thus regular clinical screening for signs and symptoms of end-organ damage (cardiac, cerebral, and peripheral vascular organs) is required. Under-treatment has been well documented in CKD populations, and thus it is imperative that practitioners recognise the risk of CVD in CKD populations, implement the usual prevention strategies, and identify unique complications of CKD which may exacerbate CVD.

Anaemia in CKD

What are the causes of anaemia in CKD?

- Anaemia of CKD is:
  - Due to a relative and an absolute iron deficiency.
  - And due to erythropoietin deficiency.
  - A decline in Hb is apparent with GFR <70mL/min/1.73m^2 in males and <50mL/min/1.73m^2 in females, and the prevalence increases as GFR declines.
  - Patients with diabetes are more likely to have anaemia of CKD for any given level of GFR.
  - Patients with polycystic kidney disease generally have well-maintained Hb until later stages of CKD, but relative declines in Hb will be noticed.

- The usual causes of anaemia in the general population should also be considered (Hb values between 85–110 are expected in those untreated individuals with eGFR <30mL/min).

What are the symptoms/consequences of anaemia in CKD patients?

- Fatigue.
- Cognitive impairment.
- Exercise intolerance.
- Exacerbation of cardiac ischaemia/cardiac failure.
- Left ventricular hypertrophy.
- Decreased quality of life (and improved quality of life noted with treatment).

What investigations should be ordered when evaluating anaemia in a CKD patient?

- Iron stores: serum iron, TIBC, transferrin saturation.
  - Ferritin is often elevated in CKD, even with iron deficiency, due to chronic inflammation and therefore, less reliable. However, if ferritin is low, this indicates iron deficiency.
- Haematology profile.
- Remember the non-kidney causes of anaemia in patients whose degree of anaemia seems out of proportion to the degree of kidney dysfunction (e.g. profound anaemia with Hb <100) in a patient with an eGFR >45mL/min).
- In the absence of clinical suspicion or suggestive history, search for other causes, and common causes such as B12 or folate deficiency is not routinely recommended.

Management of anaemia

Treat iron deficiency: target transferrin saturation >0.20.

- Start with oral iron therapy.
- May require intravenous iron if unresponsive to oral iron.

Erythropoietin-stimulating agents (ESAs):

- ◆ Only consider if iron replete and Hb <100g/L.

- ◆ Current available agents include erythropoietin alpha, erythropoietin beta, darbapoietin, and pegylated erythropoietin preparations.

  - • Similar efficacy between agents at comparable doses.

  - • Differences in the duration of action (usual dosing frequency every one to four weeks).

  - • Self-administered by subcutaneous route.

- ◆ Usually require referral to a specialist familiar with these agents for commencement.

- ◆ Regular monitoring of haemoglobin (usually monthly) and iron status (usually every three months) is required for patients on ESAs.

- ◆ Target Hb concentration currently 110–120g/L according to international consensus.

Management of mineral and bone metabolism abnormalities in CKD

What are the mineral and bone metabolism abnormalities in CKD?

- ◆ CKD affects the regulation of calcium and phosphate, which may result in secondary hyperparathyroidism and metabolic bone disease.

- ◆ More recently, attention has also focused on extraskeletal and cardiovascular complications, which may be a result of the derangement of mineral metabolism or the consequence of treatment with additional calcium or vitamin D.

- ◆ The abnormalities in CKD are summarized in Table 9.3.

What are the consequences of secondary hyperparathyroidism?

- ◆ Persistently elevated PTH levels may lead to bone changes and reduced bone integrity. These bone changes include:

  - • High turnover bone disease (osteitis fibrosa cystica).

  - • Adynamic bone disease.

Table 9.3 Abnormalities in mineral metabolism in CKD

Retention of phosphate begins early in CKD although serum phosphate remains in 'normal' range until later stages of CKD.

Reduced conversion of vitamin D into its active form (calcitriol (1,25-dihydroxyvitamin D)) due to reduced renal 1-alpha-hydroxylase activity.

Reduced serum calcium due to decreased absorption.

Hypersecretion of parathyroid hormone (PTH), an initially appropriate physiologic response to raise serum calcium (by increasing calcium reabsorption) and lower serum phosphate (by increasing renal phosphate excretion).

Progression to secondary hyperparathyroidism and development of renal osteodystrophy.

- Osteomalacia.
- Osteoporosis.

- The incidence of fractures in CKD is higher than that of the general population, thus attention to strategies to preserve normal bone turnover, mineralization, and bone and muscle strength are essential.

- Low levels of 1,25-dihydroxyvitamin D, hypocalcaemia, and hyperphosphataemia all increase PTH secretion: these abnormalities themselves have consequences (see below).

- Elevated serum phosphate is associated with increased morbidity and mortality, has been linked to symptoms such as pruritus, and has been shown in experimental models to contribute to the vascular dysfunction and calcification seen in CKD. (vascular calcification is reported to occur in 40–70% of CKD stage 4 patients).

- PTH may also be an important uraemic toxin, impacting both vascular function and cardiac structure.

What tests should be ordered to evaluate mineral and bone metabolism abnormalities in CKD?

- Serum calcium, phosphorus, PTH, albumin (a correction is required to assess the free calcium concentration if hypoalbuminaemic).

- Current recommendations would include annual measurements in stage 3; at least 3–6 monthly testing in those with stages 4 and 5. Earlier repeat measurements should be considered if levels are abnormal or treatment changes are implemented. Consideration of the age of the patient, costs of testing, and health system issues will affect test frequency.

♦ Target values include serum calcium and phosphorus in the normal laboratory range (2.2–2.5mmol/L and 0.75–1.4mmol/L, respectively). The PTH value targets are controversial at the writing of this chapter and should be discussed with nephrology experts for local guidance.

♦ At the current time, the measurement of serum 25- and 1,25-dihydroxyitamin D levels are not well standardized, despite the former being measured by many laboratories. Caution in interpretation and measurement is advised.

  • A bone biopsy is the gold standard for the diagnosis of renal bone disease, but is seldom used clinically due to the invasiveness of the procedure.

  • Bone mineral densitometry is not well standardized in CKD patients and may not be as useful in more advanced CKD. Discussion with local experts prior to the ordering of this test is recommended.

Approach to treatment

Phosphate control

♦ Should be instituted early in the course of CKD to prevent secondary hyperparathyroidism.

♦ Dietary phosphate restriction (to 800–1,000mg/day).

  • Dieticians with renal training can advise on dietary phosphate restriction while avoiding malnutrition and protein deficiency which are risks of severe phosphate restriction.

Oral phosphate binders

♦ Calcium-based agents (calcium carbonate, calcium acetate).

  • Most effective if taken with food to bind dietary phosphate before it is absorbed.

♦ Non-calcium-based binders (sevelamer, lanthanum).

  • Reserved for patients intolerant to calcium-based binders or who develop hypercalcaemia with calcium-based agents.

  • Much more expensive than calcium-based agents.

Vitamin D analogues

◆ Vitamin D deficiency is ubiquitous in the general population as well as the CKD population.

◆ Recently, an association between vitamin D deficiency, inflammation, and CVD has been suggested.

◆ Treatment with vitamin D helps suppress PTH, prevent osteoporosis, and improve muscle strength.

◆ Vitamin D is usually supplemented as either the active metabolite calcitriol (1,25-dihydroxyvitamin D) or precursors of calcitriol that use the liver for conversion to calcitriol (e.g. alphacalcidol). Several other vitamin D analogues have been developed and are in clinical use.

◆ If a patient is on traditional vitamin D supplementation (i.e. 400–1,000IU) with normal parameters of mineral metabolism in CKD stage 1–3, this should be continued and parameters monitored annually.

◆ Calcimimetics (oral agents that decrease PTH secretion by increasing the sensitivity of the calcium-sensing receptor on the parathyroid gland) and a surgical parathyroidectomy are other methods that nephrologists might consider to treat refractory hyperparathyroidism in CKD patients, but this is generally only needed in a few patients in the late stages of CKD.

Management of metabolic acidosis in CKD

◆ Metabolic acidosis (serum bicarbonate <22mmol/L) occurs due to:
  • Reduced ability of the kidney to generate new bicarbonate.
  • Continued ingestion of acid loads.

◆ The consequences of chronic metabolic acidosis, even if mild, include:
  • The potential to worsen bone disease (due to the release of calcium from bone and impaired vitamin D receptor binding).
  • The potential to cause muscle protein catabolism and lower albumin.
  • Renal stone formation (with prolonged and more severe metabolic acidosis).

- Treatment of metabolic acidosis in CKD patients can include:
  - Supplementation with exogenous alkali to keep serum bicarbonate >22mmol/L.
  - The most commonly used agent is sodium bicarbonate (given as tablets or as baking soda powder dissolved in liquid).
  - Note that calcium carbonate, often used as a phosphate binder, will raise bicarbonate levels as the carbonate is converted to bicarbonate after ingestion.

CKD and malnutrition

Prevalence and risk factors

- Common in patients with CKD and increases as kidney disease worsens (approximately 20–60% of patients with CKD stages 3–5).
- Portends a worse outcome in CKD patients.
- Risk factors for malnutrition in CKD are listed in Table 9.4 and relate to their underlying disease, kidney disease itself, or the complications of treatment.

Dietary recommendations

- The general recommendations outlined in Table 9.5 can be applied to most patients with CKD stages 3–5 (excluding patients on dialysis).

Protein requirements in CKD

- Healthy individuals require a daily protein intake of 0.6–0.75g/kg/day to avoid protein-calorie malnutrition.

Table 9.4 Risk factors for malnutrition in CKD

Factors related to their underlying disease (e.g. gastroparesis with diabetes mellitus)
Polypharmacy
Decreased taste and smell
Uraemic toxin accumulation
Decreased intestinal absorption and digestion
Metabolic acidosis causing protein catabolism
Elevated PTH level (which may promote gluconeogenesis and amino acid catabolism)
Amino acid abnormalities

Table 9.5 General dietary recommendations for CKD patients

Energy intake <60 years	35kcal/kg/day
Energy intake >60 years	30kcal/kg/day
Protein	0.8–1g/kg/day
Sodium	<2g/day
Phosphorus	<800mg/day

- The average diet provides 1g/kg/day of protein.
- In patients with CKD, poor appetite often leads to a self-imposed restriction of daily protein intake to <0.6g/kg/day and weight loss.
- Dietary protein restriction has often been recommended as a method of preventing or slowing the progression of CKD.
  - Evidence has been controversial and often conflicting.
  - Some studies have shown no difference in CKD progression, others have shown a modest reduction in urinary protein excretion.
  - Currently, there is insufficient evidence to conclude that a protein-restricted diet delays CKD progression.
- On balance, a protein-controlled diet without restriction (0.8–1g/kg/day of high biologic value protein) is recommended in CKD stages 1–3 and a restriction of 0.6–0.75 g/kg/day may be considered in CKD stages 4–5 (not on dialysis) only under the careful supervision of a dietician with close dietary counselling and monitoring of biochemical and nutritional indices to avoid malnutrition.

Vitamin supplementation

- Avoidance of specific supplements.
  - Supplementation with vitamin A is not recommended as levels are usually elevated in CKD patients and supplementation may lead to vitamin A toxicity.
  - The supplemental use of vitamin E is also not currently recommended in CKD patients due to lack of benefit noted in recent studies and potential for toxicity.
- Supplementation with water-soluble vitamins.
  - The concentration of water-soluble vitamins (B6, B12, others) are often decreased in CKD patients and special multivitamin

preparations are available for CKD patients that can correct these deficiencies without exposure to excessive vitamin A.

Assessment and monitoring of nutritional status

Serum albumin: monitor at least yearly and target the normal range.

- Note it may be unreliable in CKD patients as:
  - Serum albumin decreases with inflammation.
  - Urinary protein loss as a result of the underlying kidney disease may lead to lower serum albumin, independent of nutritional status.
- Even given these limitations, serial measurements of serum albumin in stable patients can be used as one marker of nutritional status.

Lean body mass: weigh the patient at each visit and track the percentage of weight change.

- Body mass index (BMI), skinfold thickness, and mid-arm muscle circumference can also be used to analyze body composition.
- As kidney disease progresses, lean body mass often decreases and it is an indication of progressing malnutrition and provides an indication to start renal replacement therapy (RRT).

Subjective Global Assessment (SGA) combines objective data (including disease state and weight change) with a series of questions regarding recent changes in nutritional intake.

- It provides a standard format on which to conduct a nutritional assessment and has been validated for use in dialysis patients.
- Patients are classified as well nourished, mildly malnourished/suspected malnutrition or severely malnourished.

In summary, CKD patients are at risk of malnutrition. No single marker properly reflects the nutritional status in CKD patients. Close supervision and nutritional counselling is recommended for most CKD patients, especially those on protein-restricted diets. Dietary counselling in the CKD clinic is associated with improved BP control, preservation of visceral protein stores and lean body mass, and improvements in serum phosphate, potassium, and bicarbonate. In patients with advanced CKD, progressive malnutrition and weight loss unresponsive to dietary interventions are an indication to start RRT.

Preparing CKD patients for RRT or conservative care

Individuals with progressive CKD require preparation for either RRT (dialysis or transplantation) or comprehensive conservative care. Creating and implementing these care plans is an ongoing process that takes time and often requires input from several members of the health care team working with the individual. Each modality of RRT has its strengths and limitations, and the role of the primary care provider and the CKD care team is to determine which modality is right for the individual with CKD. The different modalities should be seen as complementary and individuals may transition through many modalities during their life. Early education and optimal preparation improve outcomes, including increased length of time to ESRD, improved preemptive transplant rates, increased arteriovenous fistula (AVF) use, and increased patient survival on dialysis.

When to start planning?

- Timely preparation for RRT is important and must be weighed against the perceived chance of the individual progressing to ESRD.
  - For example, a young patient with diabetic nephropathy and persistent proteinuria and an eGFR that has gone from 70mL/min to 50mL/min over a year has a much higher risk of progression to ESRD than an 85-year old, well-controlled, hypertensive individual with a stable eGFR of 18mL/min for three years and no proteinuria.
- There is no evidence to suggest a certain level of eGFR (in the absence of complications) below which dialysis should be initiated.
- Observe patients with an eGFR <20mL/min carefully for symptoms of uraemia, metabolic complications (hyperkalaemia, acidosis), volume overload (resistant oedema, hypertension) or a decline in nutritional status that have been refractory to medical interventions. The presence of these symptoms or signs may indicate the need to start RRT.

The role of the multidisciplinary clinic

- Multidisciplinary CKD teams typically include dieticians, pharmacists, social workers, nurse clinicians and/or nurse practitioners, and nephrologists.

- Education includes lifestyle modification, dietary and medication management, modality selection and vascular access, and renal transplantation.
- Many of the anticipated benefits of CKD multidisciplinary clinics (MDC) have been confirmed in studies and are summarized in Table 9.6.
- Not all individuals with CKD require care in an MDC.
  - For example, an individual with an established cause for their CKD with a stable eGFR >30mL/min, controlled BP <130/80, controlled urinary protein excretion (PCR <100mg/mmol or ACR <60mg/mmol), and haemoglobin, calcium, phosphorus, and PTH in the normal range, then follow-up with primary care and nephrology support as needed is recommended.

Kidney transplantation

- For eligible patients, a live donor kidney transplant should be promoted as the first choice of RRT.
  - Consider if eGFR is <20mL/min along with evidence of progressive renal damage over the prior 6–12 months.
- Primary care providers can play an integral role in preparing their patient for kidney transplantation by knowing:
  - Who is eligible (there are few absolute contraindications and no absolute age cut-off).

Table 9.6 CKD multidisciplinary interventions and noted benefits

Dietary counselling: improved BP control, preservation of visceral protein stores and lean body mass, and improvements in serum phosphate, potassium, and bicarbonate
Pharmacy counselling: improved adherence to therapy in a population where polypharmacy is common
Greater use of ACEis, iron, and bicarbonate therapy
Greater likelihood of having a functioning vascular access at dialysis initiation
Improved patient's perceived health-related quality of life
Reduced mortality in some studies, but not others

- What investigations should be done while an individual is waiting on the transplant list (such as ensuring vaccinations and cardiac testing).
- Notifying the transplant programme if there have been changes in the patients' status.

Dialysis

- Current evidence suggests that both peritoneal dialysis (PD) and haemodialysis (HD) provide equivalent RRT for most patients and therefore, modality selection is based on patient preference in most cases.
- Home-based therapies (PD and home HD) are promoted for their advantages, including increased patient autonomy, increased flexibility, and reduced overall costs.
- Preparation for RRT differs, depending on the modality chosen so it is important to educate patients and encourage a modality choice before RRT is needed.
- All patients with progressive CKD should be taught to protect their non-dominant arm from venepuncture, intravenous cannulation, or BP measurements as these can reduce the quality of the veins available for AVF creation if haemodialysis is required.

Peritoneal dialysis

- An underutilized first option for many new dialysis patients (11% of the dialysis population worldwide).
- Relatively simple and less expensive than haemodialysis.
- Does not require access to the bloodstream.
- There are few contraindications to PD.
- Preparation includes the insertion of a PD catheter into the peritoneal cavity about two to four weeks before use.
- PD regimens include continuous ambulatory PD (CAPD) which involves manual daytime exchanges or automated PD (APD) which uses a machine to perform the dialysis exchanges, usually done overnight.

Haemodialysis

* The most common form of RRT in developed countries.

* The majority of patients receive HD in a facility that provides full care; however, some individuals participate in their HD care in assisted or self-care units.

* Conventional HD is provided for four hours per session, three times a week.

* Some patients dialyze at home (home HD), either for conventional amounts of time or for extended periods of time overnight (nocturnal dialysis).

Vascular access timing and planning for haemodialysis

* An AVF is the preferred access for haemodialysis as it is the most dependable access with the lowest risk of complications.

* An artificial, arteriovenous graft is a second-line option and a tunnelled haemodialysis catheter is only used as a last resort due to higher rates of local and systemic infection, central venous stenosis, thrombosis, and increased mortality.

* AVFs take a minimum of four weeks and often as long as three to six months to mature. Therefore, access planning should start **a minimum of 6–12 months before dialysis is anticipated.**

  * Timely referral to nephrology is recommended and has been associated with an increased rate of AVF use and reduced mortality.

* Vascular access planning should begin when the patient has an estimated GFR of 15–20mL/min **and evidence of progressive renal disease**.

Comprehensive conservative management

* Individuals may choose not to undergo RRT if their kidney function declines. This decision should be made after appropriate education regarding their choices and in consultation with members of the health care team (including primary care providers, nephrologists, CKD nurses, dieticians, social workers, psychologists, spiritual care workers, palliative care physicians/nurses, and appropriately trained and supervised volunteers).

- A care plan with shared decision-making that addresses the medical, psychological, and spiritual needs of the patient/family and caregivers should be developed.

- Note that often the preferences of the individual changes and frequent re-evaluation of the care plan is required to ensure it reflects a feasible set of options that aligns with the individuals' current wishes.

Conclusions

The management of patients with CKD requires a coordinated plan of care that involves the ongoing input of multiple care providers. The use of a multidisciplinary CKD clinic can help to manage the complications of CKD that require extra support, ideally leading to an engaged and educated patient ready to take an active role in maintaining their health. It is critical to ensure that all practitioners have a clear understanding of what role and responsibilities they have in the patients' care plan. This will lead to an efficient and effective treatment and will minimize the chances of medical error.

Preparation for RRT and conservative care constitute part of the spectrum of care of the complications of CKD. Ideally, these activities are best done with the collaboration of a trained team of individuals who understand the condition, the resources available to those with CKD, and how to best implement the strategies described here.

The role of the general practitioner and non-nephrology specialists is to identify individuals with CKD or at risk for CKD, and to develop a care plan and strategy to mitigate the risk of complications of the condition. Within a framework of regular CVD risk mitigation and recognizing some unique additional contributors to CKD morbidity and mortality described herein, there is a possibility that we can improve the outcomes of this population.

References

Anaemia and Mineral Metabolism

Abu–Alfa, A.K., Sloan, L., Charytan, C., Sekkarie, M., Scarlata, D., Globe, D., Audhya, P., 2008. The association of darbepoetin alfa with hemoglobin and health-related quality of life in patients with chronic kidney disease not receiving dialysis. *Current Medical Research and Opinion*, 24(4), pp.1091–100.

Alem, A.M., Sherrard, D.J., Gillen, D.L., Weiss, N.S., Beresford, S.A., Heckbert, S.R., Wong, C., Stehman–Breen, C., 2000. Increased risk of hip fracture among patients with end-stage renal disease. *Kidney International*, 58(1), pp.396–9.

Astor, B.C., Muntner, P., Levin, A., Eustace, J.A., Coresh, J., 2002. Association of kidney function with anaemia: the Third National Health and Nutrition Examination Survey (1988–1994). *Archives of Internal Medicine*, 162(12), pp.1401–8.

Block, G.A., Klassen, P.S., Lazarus, J.M., Ofsthun, N., Lowrie, E.G., Chertow, G.M., 2004. Mineral metabolism, mortality, and morbidity in maintenance hemodialysis. *Journal of the American Society of Nephrology*, 15(8), pp.2208–18.

Chertow, G.M., Raggi, P., Chasan–Taber, S., Bommer, J., Holzer, H., Burke, S.K., 2004. Determinants of progressive vascular calcification in haemodialysis patients. *Nephrology Dialysis Transplantation*, 19(6), pp.1489–96.

Coen, G., Bonucci, E., Ballanti, P., Balducci, A., Calabria, S., Nicolai, G.A., Fischer, M.S., Lifrieri, F., Manni, M., Morosetti, M., Moscaritolo, E., Sardella, D., 2002. PTH 1-84 and PTH "7-84" in the noninvasive diagnosis of renal bone disease. *American Journal of Kidney Diseases*. 40(2), pp.348–54.

Coen, G., Calabria, S., Bellinghieri, G., Pecchini, F., Conte, F., Chiappini, M.G., Ferrannini, M., Lagona, C., Mallamace, A., Manni, M., DiLuca, M., Sardella, D., Taggi, F., 2001. Parathyroidectomy in chronic renal failure: short- and long-term results on parathyroid function, blood pressure and anaemia. *Nephron*, 88(2), pp.149–55.

Drueke, T.B., Locatelli, F., Clyne, N., Eckardt, K.U., Macdougall, I.C., Tsakiris, D., Burger, H.U., Scherhag, A.; CREATE Investigators, 2006. Normalization of hemoglobin level in patients with chronic kidney disease and anaemia. *New England Journal of Medicine*, 355(20), pp.2071–84.

El-Achkar, T.M., Ohmit, S.E., McCullough, P.A., Crook, E.D., Brown, W.W., Grimm, R., Bakris, G.L., Keane, W.F., Flack, J.M.; Kidney Early Evaluation Programme, 2005. Higher prevalence of anaemia with diabetes mellitus in moderate kidney insufficiency: The Kidney Early Evaluation Programme. *Kidney International*, 67(4), pp.1483–8.

Fried, L.F., Biggs, M.L., Shlipak, M.G., Seliger, S., Kestenbaum, B., Stehman–Breen, C., Sarnak, M., Siscovick, D., Harris, T., Cauley, J., Newman, A.B., Robbins, J., 2007. Association of kidney function with incident hip fracture in older adults. *Journal of the American Society of Nephrology*, 18(1), pp.282–6.

Guerin, A.P., Pannier, B., Marchais, S.J., London, G.M., 2008. Arterial structure and function in end-stage renal disease. *Current Hypertension Reports*, 10(2), pp.107–11.

Hutchison, A.J., Whitehouse, R.W., Boulton, H.F., Adams, J.E., Mawer, E.B., Freemont, T.J., Gokal, R., 1993. Correlation of bone histology with parathyroid hormone, vitamin D3, and radiology in end-stage renal disease. *Kidney International*, 44(5), pp.1071–7.

KDOQI, 2003. Clinical practice guidelines for bone metabolism and disease in chronic kidney disease. *American Journal of Kidney Diseases*, 42(4 Suppl 3), S1–201.

KDOQI, 2007. Clinical practice guideline and clinical practice recommendations for anaemia in chronic kidney disease: 2007 update of haemoglobin target. *American Journal of Kidney Diseases*, 50(3), pp.471–530.

Lehmann, G., Stein, G., Huller, M., Schemer, R., Ramakrishnan, K., Goodman, W.G., 2005. Specific measurement of PTH (1-84) in various forms of renal osteodystrophy (ROD) as assessed by bone histomorphometry. *Kidney International*, 68(3), pp.1206–14.

Levin, A., Bakris, G.L., Molitch, M., Smulders, M., Tian, J., Williams, L.A., Andress, D.L., 2007. Prevalence of abnormal serum vitamin D, PTH, calcium, and phosphorus in patients with chronic kidney disease: results of the study to evaluate early kidney disease. *Kidney International*, 71(1), pp.31–8.

Locatelli, F., Aljama, P., Barany, P., Canaud, B., Carrera, F., Eckardt, K.U., Horl, W.H., Macdougal, I.C., Macleod, A., Wiecek, A., Cameron, S.; European Best Practice Guidelines Working Group, 2004. Revised European best practice guidelines for the management of anaemia in patients with chronic renal failure. *Nephrology Dialysis Transplantation*, 19 Suppl 2, ii1–47.

Moe, S.M., Drueke, T., Lameire, N., Eknoyan, G., 2007. Chronic kidney disease-mineral-bone disorder: a new paradigm. *Advances in Chronic Kidney Disease*, 14(1), pp.3–12.

Nasri, H., Baradaran, A., 2004. Close association between parathyroid hormone and left ventricular function and structure in end-stage renal failure patients under maintenance hemodialysis. *Bratisl Lek Listy*, 105(10–11), pp.368–73.

Pollock, C., McMahon, L., 2005. The CARI guidelines. Biochemical and haematological targets guidelines. Haemoglobin. *Nephrology*, 10 Suppl 4, S108–15.

Qi, Q., Monier–Faugere, M.C., Geng, Z., Malluche, H.H., 1995. Predictive value of serum parathyroid hormone levels for bone turnover in patients on chronic maintenance dialysis. *American Journal of Kidney Diseases*, 26(4), pp.622–31.

Revicki, D.A., Brown, R.E., Feeny, D.H., Henry, D., Teehan, B.P., Rudnick, M.R., Benz, R.L., 1995. Health-related quality of life associated with recombinant human erythropoietin therapy for predialysis chronic renal disease patients. *American Journal of Kidney Diseases*, 25(4), pp.548–54.

Sigrist, M.K., Taal, M.W., Bungay, P., McIntyre, C.W., 2007. Progressive vascular calcification over 2 years is associated with arterial stiffening and increased mortality in patients with stages 4 and 5 chronic kidney disease. *Clinical Journal of the American Society of Nephrology*, 2(6), pp.1241–8.

Singh, A.K., Szczech, L., Tang, K.L., Barnhart, H., Sapp, S., Wolfson, M., Reddan, D.; CHOIR Investigators, 2006. Correction of anaemia with epoetin alfa in chronic kidney disease. *New England Journal of Medicine*, 355(20), pp.2085–98.

Tonelli, M., Blake, P.G., Muirhead, N., 2001. Predictors of erythropoietin responsiveness in chronic hAemodialysis patients. *ASAIO Journal*, 47(1), pp.82–5.

Tonelli, M., Sacks, F., Pfeffer, M., Gao, Z., Curhan, G., 2005. Relation between serum phosphate level and cardiovascular event rate in people with coronary disease. *Circulation*, 112(17), pp.2627–33.

World Health Organization, 1994. *Indicators and strategies for iron deficiency and anaemia programmes.* Report for the WHO/UNICEF/UNU Consultation. 6–10 December 1993.

CKD and malnutrition

Akpele, L., Bailey, J.L., 2004. Nutrition counselling impacts serum albumin levels. *Journal of Renal Nutrition*, 14(3), pp.143–8.

Aparicio, M., Chauveau, P., Combe, C., 2001. Low protein diets and outcome of renal patients. *Journal of Nephrology*, 14(6), pp.433–9.

Cliffe, M., Bloodworth, L.L., Jibani, M.M., 2001. Can malnutrition in predialysis patients be prevented by dietetic intervention? *Journal of Renal Nutrition*, 11(3), pp.161–5.

Enia, G., Sicuso, C., Alati, G., Zoccali, C., 1993. Subjective global assessment of nutrition in dialysis patients. *Nephrology Dialysis Transplantation*, 8(10), pp.1094–8.

Garg, A.X., Blake, P.G., Clark, W.F., Clase, C.M., Haynes, R., Moist, L.M., 2001. Association between renal insufficiency and malnutrition in older adults: results from the NHANES III. *Kidney International*, 60(5), pp.1867–74.

Ikizler, T.A., 2005. Nutrition and kidney disease. In: A. Greenberg, ed. 2005. *Primer on kidney diseases.* San Diego: Academic Press, p.495.

Ikizler, T.A., Greene, J., Wingard, R.L., Parker, R.A., Hakim, R.M., 1995. Spontaneous dietary protein during progression of chronic renal failure. *Journal of the American Society of Nephrology*, 6(5), pp.1386–91.

Ikizler, T.A., Hakim, R.M., 1996. Nutrition in end stage renal disease. *Kidney International*, 50, pp.343–57.

KDOQI, 2000. Clinical practice guidelines for nutrition in chronic renal failure. *American Journal of Kidney Diseases*, 6(Suppl), S1–140.

Klahr, S., Levey, A.S., Beck, G.J., Caggiula, A.W., Hunsicker, L., Kusek, J.W., Striker, G., 1994. The effects of dietary protein restriction and blood-pressure control on the progression of chronic renal disease. *New England Journal of Medicine*, 330(13), pp.877–84.

Kopple, J.D., Greene, T., Chumlea, W.C., Hollinger, D., Maroni, B.J., Merrill, D., Scherch, L.K., Schulman, G., Wang, S.R., Zimmer, G.S., 2000. Relationship between nutritional status and the glomerular filtration rate: results from the MDRD study. *Kidney International*, 57(4), pp.1688–703.

Lancaster, K.J., 2004. Dietary treatment of blood pressure in kidney disease. *Advances in Chronic Kidney Disease*, 11(2), pp.217–21.

Young, G.A., Kopple, J.D., Lindholm, B., Vonesh, E.F., De Vecchi, A., Scalamogna, A, Castelnova, C., Oreopoulos, D.G., Anderson, G.H., Bergstrom, J., 1991. Nutritional assessment of continuous APD patients: an international study. *American Journal of Kidney Diseases*, 17(4), pp.462–71.

Preparing CKD patients for RRT or conservative care

Allon, M., Lockhart, M.E., Lilly, R.Z., Gallichio, M.H., Young, C.J., Barker, J., Deierhoi, M.H., Robbin, M.L., 2001. Effect of preoperative sonographic mapping on vascular access outcomes in haemodialysis patients. *Kidney International*, 60(5), pp.2013–20.

Curtis, B.M., Ravani, P., Malberti, F., Kennett, F., Taylor, P.A., Djurdjev, O., Levin, A., 2005. The short- and long-term impact of multi-disciplinary clinics in addition to standard nephrology care on patient outcomes. *Nephrology Dialysis Transplantation*, 20(1), 147–54.

Davison, S.N., Torgunrud, C., 2007. The creation of an advance care planning process for patients with ESRD. *American Journal of Kidney Diseases*, 49(1), pp.27–36.

Devins, G.M., Mendelssohn, D.C., Barre, P.E., Taub, K., Binik, Y.M., 2005. Predialysis psychoeducational intervention extends survival in CKD: a 20-year follow-up. *American Journal of Kidney Diseases*, 46(6), pp.1088–98.

Foley, R.N., Collins, A.J., 2007. End-stage renal disease in the United States: an update from the United States renal data system. *Journal of the American Society of Nephrology*, 18(10), pp.2644–8.

Goldstein, M., Yassa, T., Dacouris, N., McFarlane, P., 2004. Multidisciplinary predialysis care and morbidity and mortality of patients on dialysis. *American Journal of Kidney Diseases*. 44(4), pp.706–14.

Grassmann, A., Gioberge, S., Moeller, S., Brown, G., 2005. ESRD patients in 2004: global overview of patient numbers, treatment modalities and associated trends. *Nephrology Dialysis Transplantation*, 20(12), pp.2587–93.

Hemmelgarn, B.R., Manns, B.J., Zhang, J., Tonelli, M., Klarenbach, S., Walsh, M., Culleton, B.F., 2007. Association between multidisciplinary care and survival for elderly patients with chronic kidney disease. *Journal of the American Society of Nephrology*, 18(3), pp.993–9.

Joy, M.S., DeHart, R.M., Gilmartin, C., Hachey, D.M., Hudson, J.Q., Pruchnicki, M., Dumo, P., Grabe, D.W., Saseen, J., Zillich, A.J., 2005. Clinical pharmacists as multidisciplinary health care providers in the management of CKD: a joint opinion by the Nephrology and Ambulatory Care Practice and Research Networks of the American College of Clinical Pharmacy. *American Journal of Kidney Diseases*, 45(6), pp.1105–18.

Keith, D.S., Nichols, G.A., Gullion, C.M., Brown, J.B., Smith, D.H., 2004. Longitudinal follow-up and outcomes among a population with chronic kidney disease in a large managed care organization. *Archives of Internal Medicine*, 164(6), pp.659–63.

Knoll, G., Cockfield, S., Blydt–Hansen, T., Baran, D., Kiberd, B., Landsberg, D., Rush, D., Cole, E., 2005. Canadian Society of Transplantation: consensus guidelines on eligibility for kidney transplantation. *Canadian Medical Association Journal*, 173, S1–25.

Levin, A., Lewis, M., Mortiboy, P., Faber, S., Hare, I., Porter, E.C., Mendelssohn, D.C., 1997. Multidisciplinary predialysis programs: quantification and limitations of their impact on patient outcomes in two Canadian settings. *American Journal of Kidney Diseases*, 29(4), pp.533–40.

Lorenzo, V., Martin, M., Rufino, M., Hernandez, D., Torres, A., Ayus, J.C., 2004. Predialysis nephrologic care and a functioning arteriovenous fistula at entry are associated with better survival in incident haemodialysis patients: an observational cohort study. *American Journal of Kidney Diseases*, 43(6), pp.999–1007.

Main, J., Whittle, C., Treml, J., Woolley, J., Main, A., 2006. The development of an Integrated Care Pathway for all patients with advanced life-limiting illness: the supportive care pathway. *Journal of Nursing Management*, 14(7), pp.521–8.

Meier–Kriesche, H.U., Kaplan, B., 2002. Waiting time on dialysis as the strongest modifiable risk factor for renal transplant outcomes: a paired donor kidney analysis. *Transplantation*, 74(10), pp.1377–81.

Mendelssohn, D.C., Blake, P.G., Burkart, J., Golper, T., Oreopoulous, D., 2001. Dialysis modality distribution in the United States. *American Journal of Kidney Diseases*, 37(6), pp.1330–1.

Mendelssohn, D.C., Ethier, J., Elder, S.J., Saran, R., Port, F.K., Pisoni, R.L., 2006. Haemodialysis vascular access problems in Canada: results from the Dialysis Outcomes and Practice Patterns Study (DOPPS II). *Nephrology Dialysis Transplantation*, 21(3), pp.721–8.

Thanamayooran, S., Rose, C., Hirsch, D.J., 2005. Effectiveness of a multidisciplinary kidney disease clinic in achieving treatment guideline targets. *Nephrology Dialysis Transplantation*, 20(110), pp.2385–93.

White, C.A., Pilkey, R.M., Lam, M., Holland, D.C., 2002. Pre-dialysis clinic attendance improves quality of life among haemodialysis patients. *BMC Nephrology*, 3, p.3.

Wolfe, R.A., Ashby, V.B., Milford, E.L., Ojo, A.O., Ettenger, R.E., Agodoa, L.Y., Held, P.J., Port, F.K., 1999. Comparison of mortality in all patients on dialysis, patients on dialysis awaiting transplantation and recipients of a first cadaveric transplant. *New England Journal of Medicine*, 341(23), 1725–30.

Chapter 10

Management of dialysis and transplantation patients: perspectives for primary care

Monica Beaulieu, Jagbir Gill, and Adeera Levin

General information

In some cases, the care of patients with chronic kidney disease (CKD) culminates in the need for renal replacement therapy (RRT). RRT refers to either transitioning to dialysis or receiving a kidney transplant. The purpose of this chapter is to review the key issues to consider when providing care for patients on the various forms of dialysis or with a kidney transplant. It is beyond the scope of this chapter to give detailed advice on each and every potential clinical problem that these patients may face, but with this framework, it is hoped that the general physician/non-nephrology specialist will have an improved understanding of the complexity of care, while also appreciating the need for standard general approaches.

First and foremost, we would support and foster the importance of a good communication plan between generalists and nephrologists, irrespective of whether they are in the haemodialysis (HD) unit, peritoneal dialysis (PD) unit, or a transplant programme. Individual countries or geographic regions organize the care of patient receiving RRT differently so the generalist is encouraged to understand the organization of that system in order to ensure a good knowledge of how renal care is provided and to ensure good information flow. The establishment of bidirectional communication, including potentially formalizing a framework for shared care, may be of benefit in those locations where the expectations of the patient and the care team are for sharing of care plans, implementation, and follow-up.

The following chapter describes issues related to:

◆ The specific processes of HD, peritoneal dialysis and transplantation, and common management issues.

◆ Preventative care of patients on RRT.

◆ Diet.

◆ Common comorbidities of patients on RRT.

◆ Common drug questions with respect to avoidance of drug interactions, contraindications, and cessation.

While each of these aspects of care could lead to its own chapter, the format of this is to give a wide overview of key questions so as to encourage the participation of generalists in the care of these patients who continue to need general care providers. A list of key references is given for each of the sections for further more in-depth reading.

Overview of HD

Most patients receive HD in either a hospital or community-based facility; however, some patients perform haemodialysis in their own home. The following information about haemodialysis may be helpful to know.

◆ Haemodialysis requires reliable access to the patient's bloodstream called vascular access.

◆ Of the three types of vascular access (arteriovenous (AV) fistula, AV graft, catheter), an AV fistula is preferred due to a lower rate of complications such as infection, more reliable access to the bloodstream, and improved patient survival overall.

◆ An AV fistula is usually created at least three to four months before HD is required.

◆ Traditional HD occurs for four hours, three times per week. Patients who dialyze at home may dialyze for a longer period, several nights a week.

- Patients on HD have a 'dry weight' established, which is meant to represent their euvolaemic state (i.e. if the weight is any lower, the patient has unacceptable symptoms of hypotension, cramping, etc. on dialysis).
- Patients on HD are taught to maintain a modest fluid restriction in between HD sessions and are dialyzed to their 'dry weight' each run.

When providing primary care to a patient on HD, the following caveats are important to remember.

Vein preservation

- Vein preservation is critical because an AV fistula is needed if the patient is on HD or has the potential to ever require HD. This is important for the primary care provider to remember as a patient may not be followed by a nephrologist during the early stages of CKD. You should:
  - Minimize the use of central lines, PICC lines in HD, and pre-dialysis patients.
  - Minimize blood work or peripheral intravenous cannulations. If required, try to use the back of the patient's hands.
  - Do not take blood work or take a blood pressure (BP) on the side of an AV fistula.

Anticoagulation

- Anticoagulation is required during haemodialysis to prevent blood from clotting in the circuit and the filter. Anticoagulation generally consists of:
  - Heparin given by bolus and continuous infusion during the haemodialysis run.
  - Heparin left in the lumen of the HD catheter (for those patients using a central line for haemodialysis).

This is important for a generalist/non-nephrologist to know when identifying the causes of excess bleeding or thrombocytopaenia in a HD patient or when emergency access of the HD catheter is required such as in the emergency room. In the latter case, an amount equal to the volume of the catheter lumen (written on the catheter) should be withdrawn prior to using the catheter to avoid delivering an inadvertent bolus of heparin to the patient.

Overview of PD

PD is a home-based form of dialysis usually done by the patient or a caregiver. The following information about PD is helpful to know.

- Patients on PD have a catheter inserted into their abdomen which provides access to the peritoneal cavity.
- Dialysis solution is instilled into the peritoneal cavity, left for a period of time, and then drained back out, removing toxins and extra fluid when drained out.
- The filling and draining of the solution is either done manually (i.e. a bag of solution fills and drains using gravity) or with an automated device.
- PD schedules can either be continuous (i.e. fluid in the abdomen all the time) or intermittent (i.e. periods of the day when the abdomen is 'empty'). Table 10.1 describes the most common schedules.
- In contrast to HD, PD is usually done seven days a week.
- Patients on PD are taught to weigh themselves and adjust their PD fluids to maintain a target weight.

When providing primary care for a patient on PD, the following caveats are important to remember.

Table 10.1 Different schedules for PD

Manual	Continuous ambulatory PD (CAPD):
	Most common regimen is four exchanges with 2L instilled on each exchange.
	Some patients have no fluid at night ('dry night'), but most have a long (8–10h) night-time fill of solution.
Automated PD (APD)	Continuous cycler-assisted PD (CCPD):
	Bags are loaded at night before bed and the cycler machine is programmed to fill and empty the bags overnight.
	Some patients have no fluid during the day ('dry day'), but must have a long (14–16h) daytime fill of solution.

Maintaining residual renal function (RRF)

PD preserves RRF better than HD. This is important so remember to:
+ Avoid nephrotoxins
  + In general, patients on PD should not be prescribed nephrotoxins such as non-steroidal anti-inflammatory medications or aminoglycosides. In addition, the use of intravenous contrast dye should be avoided or used only when absolutely necessary and with appropriate measures in place to minimize contrast-induced nephrotoxicity (i.e. ensuring euvolaemia, and withholding ACEis and ARBs prior to intravenous contrast dye).

Glucose load

+ The most commonly used PD solution is glucose-based as glucose is inexpensive and acts as a good osmotic agent to pull fluid off the patient. However, some of this glucose (about 60%) is absorbed and the complications listed in Table 10.2 may be noted.

Constipation

+ Patients on PD often suffer from constipation. Even mild constipation can cause the PD catheter to malfunction, which often manifests as a failure to drain. Constipation should be treated as soon as it is noted. Appropriate agents include laxatives that do not contain magnesium or phosphorus. These include suppositories, lactulose, or saline enemas.

Transplant process

Renal patients are closely followed by the transplant team in the first few months after a transplant. The degree of follow-up thereafter will

Table 10.2 Potential complications of PD attributable to glucose-based solutions

Weight gain
Hyperlipidaemia, especially hypertriglyceridaemia
Hyperglycaemia/increased insulin requirements: insulin can be added to the PD dialysate and if glycaemic control is a concern, this should be discussed with the nephrologists.

vary depending on the medical stability of the patient and between different transplant centres. Regardless, a nephrologist should be involved in the long-term care of a transplant recipient. Therefore, in the general management of these patients, close follow-ups and discussions with the transplant nephrologist is recommended.

When providing primary care for a patient with a kidney transplant, the following questions are important to address.

How should immunosuppressive agents be managed in an 'unwell' transplant patient?

+ In transplant recipients who are acutely unwell, it is important to consider how long ago the patient had a transplant, the level of kidney function, and the impact of immunosuppression on the ongoing medical condition. These decisions should be made in consultation with local transplant experts. However, while waiting for discussion with a nephrologist, here are some general principles to consider:

  • In patients with severe sepsis or other illness, it is reasonable to reduce the dose of or hold mycophenolate mofetil (MMF).

  • Patients who have been on long-term corticosteroid therapy will benefit from stress doses of steroids in the event of acute illness.

  • Potential drug interactions with immunosuppressive agents should be considered when choosing antibiotic therapy.

  • Renal function should be monitored closely as these patients are at increased risk of developing acute kidney injury.

What is the differential diagnosis for an elevated serum creatinine/reduced GFR in a transplant patient?

+ The causes of reduced GFR in a transplant recipient is broad. Some of the most common reasons are listed in Table 10.3.

+ Early discussion with the patient's nephrologist is recommended to decide whether investigations such as a renal ultrasound or a transplant biopsy are warranted.

Table 10.3 Causes of reduced GFR in a kidney transplant recipient

Volume depletion
Calcineurin inhibitor nephrotoxicity
Acute rejection
Urinary tract obstruction
Renal artery stenosis
De novo acute kidney injury (e.g. acute tubular necrosis secondary to sepsis, drug-induced interstitial nephritis)
Virus (cytomegalovirus (CMV), polyoma)
Chronic rejection/chronic interstitial fibrosis and tubular atrophy of the transplanted kidney

What are the major causes of infection after transplant?

◆ In the first month post-transplant, most infections are related to surgical complications and include:

• Aspiration pneumonitis.

• Surgical site infections.

• Urinary tract infections.

• Infections related to indwelling vascular access catheters, urinary catheters, and surgical drains.

• Infections related to fluid collections (e.g. haematomas, lymphocoeles, pleural effusions, urinomas).

◆ After the first month, opportunistic infections, nosocomial infections, and community-acquired infections must all be considered. The most common infections due to opportunistic pathogens are listed in Table 10.4.

◆ When treating an infection in a transplant recipient, remember to review the medication profile in order to avoid potential adverse drug interactions. Antibiotics with common interactions include:

• Macrolide antibiotics (except azithromycin): increase calcineurin inhibitor (CNI) levels.

• Anti-fungals: increase CNI levels.

• Anti-tuberculous drugs: decrease CNI levels.

♦ In addition, the degree of renal function must be assessed in each patient in order to determine whether renal dosing is needed.

♦ To ensure the safe use of medications, the following steps should be taken:

  • Be aware of *all* medications that your patient is taking, including non-prescription or herbal medications.

  • Notify the transplant clinic of any prescribed medication *before* the patient begins to take it.

  • If a patient must take a medication that interacts with transplant therapy, frequent monitoring of the patient must be arranged with the transplant clinic.

Preventative care: immunizations and malignancy surveillance

Immunizations in patients on dialysis

Patients on RRT have a reduced response to vaccination, thought to be due to the immunosuppressive nature of uraemia. Despite the reduced response, patients on RRT should be vaccinated following the recommendations for the general population. In particular, there are several vaccines quite important for the dialysis population.

♦ Hepatitis B: patients on haemodialysis are routinely vaccinated against hepatitis B and their titres monitored on a regular basis. Because of the finding that the immune response to hepatitis B

Table 10.4 Major infections due to opportunistic pathogens

Pneumocystis jirovecii/carinii pneumonia (PCP)
Protozoal diseases (toxoplasmosis, leishmaniasis, and Chagas disease)
Fungal infections (histoplasmosis, coccidioidomycosis, blastomycosis)
Viral infections (HSV, HBV, HCV, BK polyomavirus, HHV-6, -7, -8 (Kaposi-associated herpes virus))
Respiratory viruses (influenza, parainfluenza, respiratory syncitial virus, adenovirus)
Tuberculosis
Gastrointestinal parasites (Cryptosporidium and Microsporidium) and viruses (CMV, rotavirus)

vaccination is more predictable at higher levels of GFR, it is better if patients who may need haemodialysis are vaccinated before they reach ESRD. This is often done by the primary care provider.

◆ Influenza and pneumococcal vaccines: although less data is available for these vaccines in patients on RRT, it is recommended that these are given as per local immunization guidelines. However, remember that the response in patients with renal failure may be less than normal, especially in the maintenance of adequate antibody titres.
  • Yearly influenza vaccines are recommended in all dialysis patients.
  • Pneumococcal vaccines are recommended in all dialysis patients.
◆ Tetanus, diphtheria, and pertussis vaccines: these should also be given as per local immunization guidelines and kept up to date.

Immunization in patients with a renal transplant

Because of the use of immunosuppressive medications, the response of a renal transplant patient to vaccines can be considered similar to a dialysis patient, often with a suboptimal antibody response and titres that fall faster than the general population. However, immunizations are important in the prevention of infection in transplant recipients.

The following points are important for the general practitioner.

◆ **Inactivated** vaccines.
  • Generally recommended as per local immunization guidelines, both before and after transplantation according to the usual schedules. These include hepatitis A and B, influenza, pneumococcus, tetanus, diphtheria, and pertussis.
◆ **Live** vaccines (includes measles, mumps and rubella, and varicella).
  • Should be **avoided after transplantation** and if needed, given before transplantation only.

Malignancy surveillance
Dialysis patients

◆ May be at higher risk of certain cancers such as urological cancers.
◆ In general, age- and gender-appropriate malignancy surveillance is recommended for dialysis patients and is often the role of the primary care provider.

- ◆ Because of the shortened life expectancy of people on dialysis, the decision for a comprehensive cancer screening must be patient-specific and include considerations of:
  - The patient's specific cancer risk.
  - The potential/eligibility for renal transplantation.

Kidney transplant patients

- ◆ Transplant recipients have a higher relative risk of certain malignancies, depending on individual risk factors and the degree of immunosuppression.
- ◆ The increased risk is attributed to immunosuppressive therapy and is most prominent for malignancies that have a viral association such as those in Table 10.5.
- ◆ In contrast, the risk for breast, lung, and prostate cancers are not higher than the general population.
- ◆ Routine cancer screening practices are recommended, but more aggressive screening may be warranted in certain cases.
  - Due to the increased risk of anogenital cancers in women after transplantation, an annual examination for anogenital lesions is recommended for women.
  - Given the increased risk of skin cancers, any suspicious skin lesions should be evaluated with a skin biopsy.

Dietary recommendations for patients on RRT

To maintain an adequate balance of protein, calories, vitamins, minerals, and fluid intake, most patients on RRT receive extensive counselling from renal dieticians. However, the following information is useful

Table 10.5 Potential malignancies post-kidney transplantation

Post-transplant lymphoproliferative disease (associated with Epstein–Barr virus)
Kaposi sarcoma associated with human herpesvirus (HHV-8)
Liver cancers (associated with hepatitis B and C)
Human papillomavirus (HPV)-associated genitourinary cancers

for the generalist/non-nephrologist to keep in mind when counselling a patient on RRT.

◆ All patients on RRT are at risk of cardiac disease, therefore a 'heart-healthy' diet is important. Sodium restriction is also important to help control BP and volume status.

◆ HD carries the most significant restrictions with respect to diet. Patients are counselled to significantly restrict:

  • Potassium and phosphorus intake (Table 10.6 lists common high potassium and high phosphorus foods).

  • Fluid intake to avoid the need to remove large amounts of fluid at each HD session.

◆ Patients on PD have similar, but often less, intensive restrictions. Of note:

  • Up to one third of PD patients may actually require potassium supplements to maintain their potassium in the normal range.

◆ All patients on dialysis must avoid **star fruit** as it contains a potentially fatal neurotoxin that patients on dialysis cannot eliminate. Mild symptoms include hiccups and nausea, but symptoms can progress to seizures and coma.

Patients with a functioning **kidney transplant** have the least dietary restrictions of all. The following information may be useful:

◆ Patients who have become accustomed to rigidly restrict their fluid intake are now encouraged to significantly increase their intake of fluids in the post-transplant period.

◆ With the restoration of normal taste and liberalization of dietary restrictions, transplant recipients will commonly gain weight post-transplantation.

  • This may be welcome in certain patients, but it is important to maintain a well-balanced diet and to consider the risks associated with excessive weight gain post-transplant.

  • Renal patients remain at high risk for cardiovascular and metabolic disease after transplantation.

- Immunosuppressive medications increase the risk of dyslipidaemia, impaired glucose tolerance, and new onset diabetes after transplantation
- Electrolyte disturbances such as hyperkalaemia may persist, mandating re-institution of certain dietary restrictions after transplantation.

Common comorbidities in patients on RRT

Cardiovascular

CVD is the most common cause of death in both dialysis and transplant patients. However, the approach to treating cardiovascular risk factors in this patient population remains controversial. The following section will describe some of these current controversies and provide advice for the generalist/non-nephrologist when managing these patients.

BP

- Most patients on dialysis are hypertensive.
- The method of measuring BP and recommended targets are controversial.
  - One suggestion is a pre-HD BP of <140/90 and a post-HD BP of <130/80.

Table 10.6 List of high potassium and high phosphorus foods

High potassium foods	Drinks: coffee (limit to 250mL/day)
	Milk
	Fruit: all dried fruit
	Bananas, mangos, grapes, pineapples
	Vegetables: tomatoes, avocadoes, spinach
	Snacks: chocolates, nuts, potato chips
High phosphorus foods	Dairy: milk, cheese, yogurt, eggs
	Meat: liver, kidney
	Fish: shellfish
	Other: cola beverages, nuts

* Avoid all salt substitutes

- Control of volume status is the mainstay of hypertensive treatment for patients on HD. Proper volume control can either normalize the BP or make it easier to control in most dialysis patients.
- Control of volume status for BP control is especially helpful in PD patients as nearly all PD patients can become normotensive with strict adherence to volume control.
- Because of the close interplay with volume status, the nephrologist usually does the monitoring and treatment of BP.

Hyperlipidaemia

- Most patients on dialysis or with kidney transplants have abnormalities of lipid metabolism, including hypertriglyceridaemia, reduced high density lipoproteins (HDL), and increased lipoprotein a.
- Although it is well known that patients with CKD are at higher cardiovascular risk, it is not known whether treating elevated cholesterol in dialysis patients reduces cardiovascular events.
- The results of two recent, large, randomized, controlled studies looking at the effect of lipid-lowering with statins in haemodialysis patients both found that:
  - Statins are generally well tolerated in haemodialysis patients.
  - Statins decrease serum cholesterol in haemodialysis patients.
  - Statins have NO effect on cardiovascular end points (death from cardiovascular causes, non-fatal MI, non-fatal stroke) in haemodialysis patients.
- As a result of the findings of these trials, the role of statin therapy in haemodialyis patients is currently unclear and should be addressed on an individual basis.
- The role of statin therapy in patients on PD has not been well studied, but is often recommended as patients on PD may have a more atherogenic lipid profile due to glucose absorption from the dialysate.

Anaemia

- Anaemia of CKD is the result of reduced renal erythropoietin production, and to a lesser extent, decreased red blood cell survival. Iron deficiency and increased risk of blood loss attenuates the anaemia of CKD.

- ◆ Almost all patients on dialysis require supplemental iron and erythropoetin-stimulating agents (ESAs).
- ◆ Iron is usually given orally if a patient is on PD and intravenously if a patient is on haemodialysis.
- ◆ Target levels of haemoglobin are between 110–120g/L.
- ◆ An acute drop in haemoglobin in dialysis patients on stable doses of iron and ESAs is *not* normal and should alert the health care provider to assess for causes of anaemia as in the general population.
  - Dialysis patients are at increased risks of gastrointestinal blood loss and this should be evaluated for closely with any acute drop in haemoglobin.

Anaemia in the kidney transplant recipient

- ◆ After a kidney transplant, erythropoietin levels begin to rise within days and quadruple within one month.
  - As a result of this, all ESAs are discontinued at the time of transplantation.
  - The persistence of anaemia at one year post-transplant is associated with poor outcomes, including an increased risk of graft loss.
  - See Table 10.7 for common reversible causes of anaemia after transplantation.
  - There are limited data guiding the use of ESA in transplantation, but targets utilized in CKD should be employed. Blood transfusions

Table 10.7 Common reversible causes of anaemia after transplantation

Immunosuppressive agents	Azathioprine and MMF are myelosuppressive agents and may result in anaemia along with leukopaenia and thrombocytopaenia.
	Haemolytic-uraemic syndrome/thrombotic thrombocytopaenic purpura (HUS/TTP) secondary to CNIs and sirolimus should be considered in patients with microangiopathic haemolytic anaemia.
Antibiotics	Co-trimoxazole
Anti-viral agents	Valganciclovir
ACEis	
Viral infections	CMV, PV B19

should be avoided, if possible, and iron deficiency needs to be aggressively managed with iron supplementation.

Mineral metabolism

◆ CKD leads to hyperphosphataemia, hypocalcaemia, low activated vitamin D levels, and elevated PTH which is initially appropriate as this will lower phosphate and raise calcium.

◆ After time, PTH secretion becomes inappropriate and leads to CKD-mineral and bone disorder (CKD-MBD).

◆ Most patients on dialysis are on supplemental calcium and activated vitamin D.

◆ Calcium is also often used as a phosphate binder in patients on dialysis.
  • When oral calcium is given at the start of a meal, it acts as an effective and inexpensive phosphate binder.
  • When calcium is given between meals or at bedtime, it provides supplemental calcium.

◆ Patients on dialysis are at risk of osteoporosis in addition to traditional forms of CKD-MBD. However, the following caveats are important to remember.
  • Traditional methods of diagnosing osteoporosis such as dual-energy X-ray absorptiometry (DEXA) are not reliable in patients on dialysis and should not be used.
  • Diagnosing osteoporosis requires the exclusion of the other forms of CKD-MBD which may require specialized, biochemical testing or bone biopsy.
  • The role of bisphosphonates for patients on dialysis is unclear and they are generally not recommended for this patient population.

◆ After successful transplantation, normalization of serum phosphate, calcium, vitamin D, and PTH is expected.
  • However, persistent hyperparathyroidism is observed in 30–50% of patients after kidney transplantation, and may result in hypercalcaemia or hypophosphataemia, requiring treatment.

Diabetes

Diabetes may often be managed by the generalist/non-nephrologist. The following is important to remember.

- When using oral hypoglycaemics:
  - Certain sulfonylureas (e.g. glyburide) should be avoided in renal failure as they have the potential to accumulate. Gliclazide or glipizide are preferred as they do not accumulate.
  - Biguanides such as metformin must be avoided in dialysis patients due to the risk of lactic acidosis.
- When using insulin:
  - Insulin requirements will generally decrease as pre-dialysis renal failure progresses (due to decreased insulin degradation). Some patients may even be able to come off insulin when the GFR becomes severely compromised (i.e. <20mL/min).
  - Once on dialysis, insulin requirements may increase, especially on PD as a significant amount of the glucose used in the dialysis solution is absorbed.
  - Diabetic patients on PD are often taught to inject insulin directly into their PD dialysate.

In a diabetic patient, post-kidney transplant:

- Insulin requirements may increase post-transplantation due to:
  - Increased appetite, increased intake of carbohydrates.
  - Immunosuppressive medications may contribute to further impaired glucose tolerance or even the development of new onset diabetes (especially corticosteroids, tacrolimus, and sirolimus).
  - In many instances, the altered glycaemic state may be transient, but close follow-up is wise given the anticipated fluctuations in glycaemic control after transplantation.

Depression

- Depression is common in the dialysis population.
- In many centres, dialysis patients are followed by a renal social worker who may provide useful collateral information, both for the nephrologists and the primary care provider.

- Depression must be distinguished from under-dialysis as the symptoms (such as anorexia and failure to thrive) may be similar for the two conditions.
- The pharmacologic treatment of depression is similar to that of the general population.
  - Selective serotonin reuptake inhibitors are generally safe.

Common drug questions in dialysis and transplantation

What if a kidney transplant patient misses a dose of immunosuppression?

- If a single dose of either a CNI or MMF is missed, the dose should be taken at that time and regular dosing should resume. For example, if a patient misses their morning dose and remembers in the afternoon, the morning dose should be taken then (in the afternoon) followed by their regularly scheduled evening dose.

What are the most common drug interactions with cyclosporine and tacrolimus?

- Interactions which increase cyclosporine or tacrolimus levels.
  - The following liver enzyme inhibitors may increase cyclosporine or tacrolimus levels by more than 100%: cimetidine, erythromycin, clarithromycin and other macrolide antibiotics, diltiazem, ketoconazole, metoclopramide, metronidazole, verapamil, and heavy or binge alcohol use.
- Interactions which decrease cyclosporine or tacrolimus levels.
  - The following liver enzyme inducers can increase cyclosporine or tacrolimus metabolism, causing sub-therapeutic levels: anticonvulsants such as carbamazepine, phenobarbital, phenytoin, and anti-tuberculous agents such as isoniazid and rifampin. Large intravenous doses of co-trimoxazole have also been reported to decrease levels.
- Drugs which enhance cyclosporine or tacrolimus nephrotoxicity.
  - Drugs such as the aminoglycoside antibiotics (gentamicin, tobramycin, amikacin, etc.), aciclovir, amphotericin B, melphalan, all non-steroidal anti-inflammatory drugs (NSAIDs) have additive nephrotoxicity.

- ◆ Interactions which increase levels of concomitant drugs.
  - • Cyclosporine or tacrolimus may inhibit the metabolism of other drugs and increase levels of drugs such as digoxin. They can also increase the level of certain statins (atorvastatin, simvastatin, lovastatin), increasing the risk of rhabdomyolysis.

What is the interaction between azathioprine and allopurinol?

- ◆ Azathioprine is a common immunosuppressant used both in kidney transplant patients (especially those who have received a transplant >5–10 years ago) and in patients with autoimmune conditions.
- ◆ Allopurinol should NEVER be prescribed to someone receiving azathioprine except as a last resort and with careful monitoring.
- ◆ Allopurinol inhibits the metabolism of azathioprine metabolites, leading to potentially **life-threatening marrow suppression**. Acute gout attacks are best treated with colchicine. Avoid the use of NSAIDs. If gout attacks are recurrent, the transplant clinic will likely commence allopurinol use with marked adjustment of azathioprine dose and careful laboratory monitoring.

Can I use nitrofurantoin to treat a urinary tract infection (UTI) in a dialysis patient?

- ◆ Nitrofurantoin should not be used at all in dialysis patients. The drug needs an adequate GFR to reach effective concentrations in the urinary tract.
- ◆ In addition, toxic metabolites of nitrofurantoin may accumulate.

Which patients on RRT need to avoid intravenous contrast?

In patients with CKD, intravenous contrast is generally avoided or minimized due to the risk of contrast-induced nephrotoxity. For patients on RRT, the following caveats apply.

- ◆ If a patient is on HD, in general, one does not have to worry about the risk of nephrotoxity from intravenous contrast. However, remember that intravenous contrast, depending on the volume used, may provide a fluid bolus and may require haemodialysis afterward if the patient becomes volume-overloaded.

- If a patient is on PD, the aim is to preserve residual renal function and intravenous contrast should be minimized or avoided, except if the patient has no renal function (no urine output) left at all.

- If a patient has received a kidney transplant, the risk of intravenous contrast depends on the degree of renal function. Therefore, patients with a relatively normal kidney function may safely receive intravenous contrast. However, the usual precautions to prevent contrast nephropathy (maintain euvolaemia ± intravenous hydration, holding ACEis/ARBs) should be taken.

Can I use NSAIDs in dialysis patients? Is there a difference between cyclooxygenase-2 selective (COX-2) and traditional non-selective NSAIDs with respect to renal risk?

- NSAIDs can be used in dialysis patients who do not have residual renal function remaining. Once again, NSAIDs are generally avoided in PD patients because of the risk of compromising their residual renal function.

- There is no difference between non-selective NSAIDs and COX-2 inhibitors with respect to the potential for renal toxicity.

Why is my dialysis patient on furosemide?

- When a patient starts HD, their diuretics, including furosemide, are usually withdrawn when a patient loses urine output. They may be continued as long as there is residual urine output in an effort to minimize the amount of fluid that has to be removed by the HD machine.

- For patients on PD, diuretics, including furosemide, are often continued indefinitely to maintain urine output and permit the liberalization of fluid intake.

- For PD patients, often large doses of oral furosemide (e.g. 250mg/day) are required to maintain or increase urine output. It does not appear that the use of diuretics in this situation improves or worsens residual renal function, but may reduce the amount of high glucose exchanges that are required on PD.

Conclusion

The care of patients on dialysis or with a kidney transplant is complex and multifaceted. This chapter provides answers to some of the most frequent questions asked by generalists/non-nephrologists.

There is often little communication between the providers that care for this patient population. Nephrologists, primary care providers, and other non-nephrologist specialists should communicate with each other and their patients and identify the services that should be provided by their family physician or their nephrologist. This will avoid the possible omission or duplication of services or confusing messaging to the patient.

References

Abu-Alfa, A.K., Burkart, J., Piraino, B., Pulliam, J., Mujais, S., 2002. Approach to fluid management in peritoneal dialysis: a practical algorithm. *Kidney International Supplement*, 81, pp.S8–16.

Choudhury, D., Luna–Salazar, C., 2008. Preventive health care in chronic kidney disease and end-stage renal disease. *Nature Clinical Practice Nephrology*, 4(4), pp.194–206.

Fellstrom, B.C., Jardine, A.G., Schmieder, R.E., Holdaas, H., Bannister, K., Beutler, J., Chae, D.W., Chevaile, A., Cobbe, S.M., Gronhagen–Riska, C., De Lima, J.J., Lins, R., Mayer, G., McMahon, A.W., Parving, H.H., Remuzzi, G., Samuelsson, O., Sonkodi, S., Sci, D., Suleymanlar, G., Tsakiris, D., Tesar, V., Todorov, V., Wiecek, A., Wuthrich, R.P., Gottlow, M., Johnsson, E., Zannad, F.; AURORA Study Group, 2009. Rosuvastatin and cardiovascular events in patients undergoing haemodialysis. *New England Journal of Medicine*, 360(14), pp.1395–407.

Gunal, A.I., Duman, S., Ozkahya, M., Toz, H., Asci, G., Akcicek, F., Basci, A., 2001. Strict volume control normalizes hypertension in peritoneal dialysis patients. *American Journal of Kidney Diseases*, 37(3), pp.588–93.

Holley, J.L., 2007. Screening, diagnosis, and treatment of cancer in long-term dialysis patients. *Clinical Journal of the American Society of Nephrology*, 2(3), pp.604–10.

Medcalf, J.F., Harris, K.P., Walls, J., 2001. Role of diuretics in the preservation of residual renal function in patients on continuous ambulatory peritoneal dialysis. *Kidney International*, 59(3), pp.1128–33.

Miller, P.D., 2009. Diagnosis and treatment of osteoporosis in chronic renal disease. *Seminars in Nephrology*, 29(2), pp.144–55.

Piraino, B., Bailie, G.R., Bernardini, J., Boeschoten, E., Gupta, A., Holmes, C., Kuijper, E.J., Li, P.K., Lye, W.C., Mujais, S., Paterson, D.L., Fontan, M.P., Ramos, A., Schaefer, F., Uttley, L.; ISPD Ad Hoc Advisory Committee, 2005. Peritoneal dialysis-related infections recommendations. *Peritoneal Dialysis International*, 25(2), pp.107–31.

Wanner, C., Krane, V., Marz, W., Olschewski, M., Mann, J.F., Ruf, G., Ritz, E.; German Diabetes and Dialysis Study Investigators, 2005. Atorvastatin in patients with type 2 diabetes mellitus undergoing haemodialysis. *New England Journal of Medicine*, 353(3), pp.238–48.

Zimmerman, D.L., Selick, A., Singh, R., Mendelssohn, D.C., 2003. Attitudes of Canadian nephrologists, family physicians and patients with kidney failure toward primary care delivery for chronic dialysis patients. *Nephrology Dialysis Transplantation*, 18(2), pp.305–9.

Index